"Integrating their shared experiences, the authors, Miri Keren as an infant psychiatrist and Suzi Tortora as a dance/movement therapist, have put together an extraordinarily valuable text focused on the impact of serious medical illnesses on the development of very young children. Particularly important is the emphasis throughout the book on how very young children's development, both healthy and/or dysfunctional, is fundamentally shaped by nonverbally based physiological, sensory-motor, and affective interchanges between infants and their caregivers, interchanges that are internalized and become deeply "embodied" in the child's psyche. Building on this fundamental aspect of early development, the authors provide detailed descriptions of the mechanisms underlying young children's vulnerability to medical procedures and the potential immediate and long-term effects, the ways in which parents and medical personnel can help to reduce these potential traumatic effects, and rich descriptions of clinically effective nonverbal dance-movement techniques involving both child and caregiver. This richness of material will apply not only in work with seriously ill young children but with any young child who has experienced trauma. A special treat for every reader, not just those who work with the medically ill but any caregiver of very young children, will be the tables and appendices that describe the huge range of nonverbally based observations that caregivers can utilize to read young children's physical, mental, and emotional states."

Theodore Gaensbauer, *M.D, Clinical Professor,*
Child and Adolescent Psychiatry, University of
Colorado Health Sciences Center, Aurora, Colorado

"Drs. Tortora and Keren offer a very accessible volume here, contributing to the maturation of medical dance/movement therapy (DMT) with specialized applications for this population. The authors' vivid descriptions of clinical sessions are a fabulous introduction to DMT for the reader unfamiliar with this mind–body integrated creative arts therapy discipline. Professional clinicians and graduate students will get close-up insights to how seasoned, intuitive, and expert therapists go about this sensitive, essential work on a moment-to-moment basis. Educators will appreciate how each well-referenced chapter can stand on its own. Theoretically rooted in development, trauma, embodiment, intersubjectivity, and regulation theories and research, integrated with practical models for pediatrics and DMT, the book exemplifies the interdisciplinarity that potentiates all medical DMT and indeed, all good health care delivery."

Sherry Goodill, *Ph.D., BC-DMT, NCC, LPC,*
Clinical Professor, Department of Creative Arts Therapies,
College of Nursing and Health Professions,
Drexel University, Philadelphia

T0373560

"To begin to understand how significant illness affects infants and children is quite daunting – this work by Dr. Tortora and Dr. Keren is excellent in exploring the intersection of experience and development with the added important insight of how dance/movement therapy can be used to intervene in these situations. I'm glad to know this work now exists, strengthening our understanding of the power of dance and movement."

Nirupa Raghunathan, *M.D., Director, Pediatric Integrative Medicine, Integrative Medicine Service, Department of Medicine, Memorial Sloan Kettering Center, New York*

Dance/Movement Therapy for Infants and Young Children with Medical Illness

This book presents dance/movement therapy as a window into the emotional and internal experience of a baby with a medical illness, within the context of treating the whole family system and using the DC: 0–5™ as the basis for formulating the clinical situation.

This book fills a gap in the literature, bringing a variety of fields together including infant mental health, infant and child psychiatry, nonverbal movement analysis, and the creative arts therapies. Grounded in a biopsychosocial perspective, dance/movement therapy is introduced as the main treatment modality, using nonverbal expression as a means of communication, and dance and music activities as intervention tools, to support the child and family. Vignettes are presented throughout the book both during and years after the medical experience, taking into consideration the subtle and more obvious effects of illness on the child's later emotional, social, and behavioral development. They illustrate the expertise of the authors as infant mental health professionals, drawing upon their work in hospitals and private practices, and highlight their unique perspectives and years of collaboration.

This exciting new book is essential reading for clinicians and mental health professionals working with infants and their families.

Suzi Tortora, Ed.D., BC-DMT, LCAT, a board-certified dance/movement therapist and specialist in the field of infant mental health and development, has a private dance/movement psychotherapy practice in New York City and Cold Spring, New York. She is the International Medical Creative Arts Spokesperson for the Andréa Rizzo Foundation and senior dance/movement therapist at Integrative Medicine Service, Memorial Sloan Kettering Cancer Center, NYC.

Miri Keren, M.D., a child and adolescent psychiatrist, is Clinical Assistant Professor Emeritus at Tel Aviv University, a clinical and research consultant at the Early Childhood Outpatient clinic of Ziv Bar Ilan University, Beit Izi Shapira Center for disabled infants and toddlers, and at the Failure to Thrive unit of the Schneider Hospital for Sick Children. She is the former president of the World Association for Infant Mental Health and Chair of the World Psychiatric Association Perinatal Section.

DMT with Infants, Children, Teens, and Families

Series Editor: Suzi Tortora, Ed.D, BC-DMT, LCAT, a board-certified dance/movement therapist and specialist in the field of infancy mental health and development, has a private dance/movement psychotherapy practice in New York City and Cold Spring, New York.

DMT with Infants, Children, Teens, and Families provides a detailed overview of all the applications of dance/movement therapy nationally and internationally, from its ancient roots in tribal healing rituals to its current uses in medical settings, schools, and private practice to support families and their children, including those with medical illness, generalized anxiety disorders, sensory processing disorders, autism spectrum disorders, eating disorders, trauma, multigenerational trauma, identity issues, and work with immigrants, refugees, people of color, and underserved populations.

The international authors contributing chapters to this series include early innovators, established leaders and young professionals bringing new perspectives to working with children and families. These diverse voices build a discussion about the use of dance to heal children using a multicultural lens that is sensitive and inclusive, with full awareness of the underlying influences power, privilege, and oppression have on servicing these populations. Each book includes theoretical/methodological and empirical chapters with many vignettes illustrating DMT in action, in addition to discussing the most prominent innovators in the field both historically and currently.

Dance/Movement Therapy for Infants and Young Children with Medical Illness
Treating Somatic and Psychic Distress
Suzi Tortora and Miri Keren

For more information about this series, please visit www.roughtledge.com/ DMT-with-Infants-Children-Teens-and-Families/book-series/DMTWICTAF

Dance/Movement Therapy for Infants and Young Children with Medical Illness

Treating Somatic and Psychic Distress

Suzi Tortora and Miri Keren

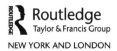
Routledge
Taylor & Francis Group

NEW YORK AND LONDON

Designed cover image by Grant Collier

First published 2023
by Routledge
605 Third Avenue, New York, NY 10158

and by Routledge
4 Park Square, Milton Park, Abingdon, Oxon, OX14 4RN

Routledge is an imprint of the Taylor & Francis Group, an informa business

Library of Congress Cataloging-in-Publication Data
Names: Tortora, Suzi, author. | Keren, Miri, author.
Title: Dance/movement therapy for infants and young children
   with medical illness: treating somatic and psychic distress/
   Suzi Tortora, Ed.D., BC-DMT, LCAT, Miri Keren, M.D.
Description: First edition. | New York, NY: Routledge, 2023.
   Series: DMT with infants, children, teens, and families | Includes
   bibliographical references and index.
Identifiers: LCCN 2022030071 (print) | LCCN 2022030072 (ebook) |
   ISBN 9780367681869 (hbk) | ISBN 9780367352608 (pbk) | ISBN
   9781003134800 (ebk)
Subjects: LCSH: Dance therapy for children.
Classification: LCC RJ505.D3 T67 2023 (print) | LCC RJ505.D3
   (ebook) | DDC 615.8/5155083—dc23/eng/20220809
LC record available at https://lccn.loc.gov/2022030071
LC ebook record available at https://lccn.loc.gov/2022030072

ISBN: 978-0-367-68186-9 (hbk)
ISBN: 978-0-367-35260-8 (pbk)
ISBN: 978-1-003-13480-0 (ebk)

DOI: 10.4324/9781003134800

Typeset in Garamond
by Apex CoVantage, LLC

Access the Support Material: www.routledge.com/9780367352608

In memory of Andréa Rizzo, whose spirit graces every one of these pages, and in dedication to Susan Rizzo Vincent, Andréa's mom, who took Dréa's vision and made it a reality.

Contents

Tables

Figures

Foreword

For infants and very young children experiencing grave and life-threatening illnesses, the world can be inhabited by pain, distress, uncertainty, and sometimes the terror of aloneness, especially when parents and others may feel unable to connect and engage with the child. This unique book, authored by Dr. Miri Keren and Dr. Suzi Tortora, both of whom I am privileged to know through our mutual connections with the World Association for Infant Mental Health, provides a vibrant and comprehensive rationale, pathway, and methodology for reaching out to enter the world of the distressed infant or young child, providing real therapeutic opportunities.

During my long career as an infant psychiatrist in a pediatric hospital setting, I have seen many young children experience considerable pain and distress due to illness and necessary but sometimes severe medical trauma. Keren and Tortora are among the few clinicians who have researched and informed us about the impacts of severe and chronic illness upon infants and preschoolers, especially those who endure long and frequent hospitalizations with concomitant medical trauma. For many years, I have been inspired by the depth of Keren and Tortora's understanding of the medically traumatized infant, and by their creative approaches to psychotherapy to alleviate infant and parent distress.

Major advances in the surgical, medical, and nursing care of young children with life-threatening disorders such as childhood cancers, congenital cardiac anomalies, and gastrointestinal disorders, including short gut syndrome, mean that children who may not have survived in an earlier era can now survive through childhood. But they often require intensive, prolonged, and frequently intrusive and painful treatments. As a result, practitioners in the field of child mental health have had to develop and adapt infant and family interventions to support these patients and their carers.

Infants comprise more than 10 percent of children who present with pediatric cancer. Researchers in related fields have stressed the importance of approaching the care of children experiencing cancer through the lens of post-traumatic stress, which affects the child and the family (Kazak & Baxt, 2007). Without attuned therapeutic intervention, more than 25 percent of infants and parents are likely to suffer significant short-term and long-term post-traumatic stress symptoms, which adversely affect much of a young child's early development.

Cardiac anomalies occur in approximately 1 percent of births. For parents whose babies are hospitalized for cardiac surgery, the rates of acute-traumatic stress symptoms are as high as 40 percent of mothers and up to 25 percent of fathers, half of whom still have these distressing symptoms a year later (Franich-Ray et al., 2013).

Now we have ways of identifying very young children who also experience post-traumatic stress syndrome because of their illness and treatment. To effectively reach these patients, we need techniques and methodologies that enable us to sensitively enter their distressed inner worlds. With this book, Keren and Tortora build on the work of Donald Winnicott, Daniel Stern, and many others who have led us straight into the mind of the infant and very young child.

This is why this book is so important. It is an amazing collaboration between an infant psychiatrist, Keren, and a dance/movement therapist, Tortora, two psychotherapists who help us enter the emotional world of the very sick young child and their parents. It is also a collaboration between the field of early interactional neurodevelopment and infant mental health and that of dance/movement therapy, led by the authors, talking and moving as if in a dance together. This is a book in which the importance of the integration of developmental psychopathology, science, and therapeutic compassion is made abundantly clear.

The clinical science of a human infant's emotional, social, regulatory, and relationship development, particularly the infant's psychophysiological response to trauma, is thoroughly enunciated by Keren throughout this book, carefully interdigitated with vivid clinical vignettes and substantiated research. Tortora demonstrates how the "preverbal" infant does have language and communicates through her body. Instead of articulate spoken words, she expresses herself through the sound of her voice; through her gaze; through hands, feet, and whole-body movements; and exquisitely timed body-to-body, person-to-person interactions. This capacity for intentional communication by infants starts at birth (Trevarthen, 1998).

The other key component of the baby's language is his capacity for play, even when very ill. Dance/movement psychotherapy can take us into this world of interpersonal communication from the very beginning. Even in the face of severe illness and possible death, it is important for the therapeutic network around young children and their parents to reinforce sensitive, attuned relationships and secure attachments. Worldwide, there have been amazing therapeutic developments that draw on dance, music, drama, and other creative arts to provide young children in the hospital with opportunities to express their feelings, and to feel in charge of their own bodies and relationships despite serious illness. Using the underpinning concept of "Embodied Parenting," Tortora describes how parents can respond to their baby's nonverbal cues, and how the baby can read the parents' communicative intention. Even in a hospital, the therapeutic dance ensues. Tortora describes ten components of her DANCE assessment tool, and from these components, we can draw inspiration and direction for the dance interaction in our day-to-day in-hospital work with infants and parents.

I was privileged to meet an 18-month-old boy and his mother after a necessary cardiothoracic surgical intervention, when he was found to have significant weakness over the left side of his body because he'd had a stroke. It wasn't clear how his recovery might progress, but my colleague and I joined him and his mother in conversation, at a measured distance. While we spoke, the boy gazed very intently and anxiously at us, as if to make sure we weren't going to cause him distress. After a little while, he seemed less anxious, and we engaged in some play with a tuneful rattle. He could not move his left side, but with his right forearm, despite the bandages and a splint that held his intravenous in place, he joined in our game, awkwardly but with purpose, moving his arm to firmly hit and sound off an array of bells on a handle that I placed within his reach. There was a real musicality to the rhythm of his arm movements and the resulting sound as he triggered the bells. His right leg moved as well, and he let me touch his toes while we spoke. He repeated this game over and over, his face softening, his expression lightening, almost becoming a smile on several occasions. The boy tenaciously held my gaze throughout and seemed very pleased and proud of what he could do to the bells with his arm and our connectedness. I think his mother, who had smiled, was also proud.

As my colleague and I reviewed the interaction with the boy, the DANCE assessment tool provided a clear framework for us to better understand what had been happening: how he moved his body; how he responded to our vocal and physical entreaties, and our touch. We had seen him enter into the rhythm of the interaction and our "co-regulated" game. Nestled comfortably and safely in his mother's arms, he seemed pleased that he could use his right arm. The game we played brought us closer within the "embraced space," a connection within interpersonal contact that he might otherwise have experienced as threatening.

Although the infant and young child experiencing a serious or life-threatening illness may specifically require the immense talents of a dance/movement psychotherapist, there is so much we can all take from Keren and Tortora's work into moment-to-moment interactions with such stressed babies and parents. We clinicians can use the fluid, interactional qualities of dance and musicality ourselves in how we speak, respond, hold, touch, and are present with the child and parents, all while being empowered to initiate seriously playful interaction. Our task is to balance the gravity of the situation for the very young child facing severe illness with that of keeping alive the child's spiritedness and human engagement.

Associate Professor Campbell Paul
Consultant Infant Psychiatrist
The Royal Children's and Royal Women's
Hospitals and the University of Melbourne
President of the World Association for Infant Mental Health

References

Franich-Ray, C., Bright, M. A., Anderson, V., Northam, E., Cochrane, A., Menahem, S., & Jordan, B. (2013). Trauma reactions in mothers and fathers after their infant's cardiac surgery. *Journal of Pediatric Psychology*, *38*(5), 494–505. https://doi.org/10.1093/jpepsy/jst015

Kazak, A. E., & Baxt, C. (2007). Families of infants and young children with cancer: A post-traumatic stress framework. *Pediatric Blood & Cancer*, *49*(S7), 1109–1113.

Trevarthen, C. (1998). The concept and foundations of infant intersubjectivity. In S. Bråten (Ed.), *Intersubjective communication and emotion in early ontogeny*. Cambridge University Press.

Acknowledgments

The development of the work described throughout this book began in 2002, when I, Suzi Tortora, was encouraged to apply to start a pediatric dance/movement therapy program at Memorial Sloan Kettering Cancer Center (MSK) in New York City. This new program, the first of its kind for MSK, was established with funds raised by the nonprofit Andréa Rizzo Foundation, then only several months old. But the genesis of the idea for a program was years before that, through Andréa Rizzo, a gifted dancer, special educator, and herself a survivor of childhood cancer. It had been her dream to give back to MSK, the place where she was healed as a baby. The untimely and tragic loss of Dréa, and the deep love from her family and friends, became the impetus to start the foundation and bring life to her passionate dream. Now, so many years later, Dréa's Dream, a dance/movement program specifically for children with cancer and special needs, is thriving at MSK and hospitals and schools across the United States. My profound thanks go to Dréa's Dream founder and president Susan Rizzo Vincent; countless volunteers, friends, and family members for their unwavering support and dedicated work; and to all the dancers, dance schools, and others who raise and provide funds to support this organization. Following their lead, a portion of the proceeds from this book will go to the Andréa Rizzo Foundation (www.dreasdream.org/).

The opportunity to start a medical dance/movement therapy program at MSK Kids, the pediatric oncology program at MSK, has been an honor and privilege that no words can truly convey. My work at MSK Kids has been fueled by the commitment and passion of doctors, nurses, the pediatric administration, psychiatry, child life specialists, integrative medicine practitioners, and all the staff, who give so much of themselves each day. Unfortunately, there is not enough room here to name every individual, but the following people have been especially instrumental in supporting the dance/movement therapists as we work together each day: Latisha Jones was the first nurse to invite me to join her work with a patient and his family in distress during a treatment; pediatric oncologist and researcher Dr. Nai-Kong Cheung was an early advocate of our work in helping pediatric patients and their families during immunotherapy treatments; pediatric oncologist Dr. Brian Kushner's spirited participation in our play turns any treatment into a dance party, immediately putting the patient and family at ease; Dr. Shakeel Modak, whose understanding of the value of this practice is evident in the opportunities he has given me to present the work to the medical team, and his introduction and recommendation of our support to families starting immunotherapy treatments; and all the multiteam discussions and collaborations across disciplines with child life specialist Jessica Anenberg, psychologist Dr. Laura Cimini, and psychiatrist Dr. Julia Kearney who have been instrumental in supporting our youngest patients and their families.

I am also indebted to our team of extraordinary integrative medicine practitioners: chief of integrative medicine Dr. Jun Mao's positive energy encourages all of us to continue to be innovative; Eva Pendleton, associate director of integrative medicine, has been my manager and friend, offering guidance with kindness and clarity; Dr. Nirupa Raghunathan, director of pediatric integrative medicine, always finds time to discuss treatment strategies and stimulates our whole team effort; music therapists Karen Popkin and Holly Mentzer, both friends and colleagues, whose spontaneous, live musical creations add a sensitive and thoughtful element to our co-treatments; Jane Greene, massage therapist and integrative medicine program coordinator, for her always thoughtful conversations; Dr. Jocelyn Shaw, the first dance therapy intern at MSK Kids, who then became my dance therapy colleague, helping to build the dance/movement therapy program in the early years; and Jennifer Whitley, my current dance therapist colleague, whose brightness, warmth, skill, and innovation make her an invaluable asset to all our programs at integrative medicine. I also thank my longtime friend and colleague, dance therapist Dr. Nancy Beardall, who has been a sounding board for all of my ideas during my whole career.

This book would not have been possible without the trust of all the young children and families Miri Keren and I have treated. We offer a special acknowledgment to each one of them, from the more than 40 years we have been privileged to work in medical and private clinical settings, with families from around the world. Finally, but not least of all, we thank our colleagues, friends, and family members who have taken the time to read many versions of our manuscript: Dr. Theodore Gaensbauer, whose advice, skill, and deep knowledge of trauma and young children have been invaluable throughout our writing process; Dr. Campbell Paul, who has provided sincere and generous support of our work, including the foreword to this book; Paul Bonnar, for his abiding editing, tech, and moral support; and Grant Collier, multimedia artist, whose beautiful and sensitive eye has added heart to our images. And, of course, our thanks go to Amanda

Savage and everyone at Routledge for patiently guiding us through the publishing process.

The dance/movement therapy work at MSK is supported in part by grants from the National Cancer Institute/National Institutes of Health (P30-CA008748) and the Andréa Rizzo Foundation, which funds the Dréa's Dream dance therapy program in hospitals and schools throughout the country.

Introduction

Daniella, age nine months, is reeling. Screaming and thrashing her tense body to and fro, she is protesting, as best as she can, the attempts of her two nurses to draw yet another blood sample. Mom is at her bedside, talking in a controlled yet anxious manner, trying to coax Daniella to calm down. Time is running out. This blood needs to be drawn now and, after their third attempt, the nurses are losing options because Daniella's small veins keep collapsing. The tension in the room is palpable. I enter at this moment, and Mom and the nurses look at me with relief. I know Daniella and her mother well, for we have been dancing together since they first started treatment for medulloblastoma three months ago. After quickly assessing the situation, I put on Daniella's favorite song, "Twinkle, Twinkle, Little Star." Mom starts to sing along as she picks up Daniella, rocking side to side. We all join in, gently swaying our bodies, quietly singing too. This dancing-lullaby interlude resets the room. As Daniella settles, snuggling into Mom's arms, the nurses are now able to carry out the procedure smoothly.

This opening vignette describes a typical dance/movement therapy (DMT) intervention used to support a parent and her infant with complex medical needs, while enabling the nurses to complete a medical procedure. This level of collaboration between the patient, family, and medical team is very common in the pediatric oncology setting where Tortora works, and DMT is part of integrative medicine holistic health services.

Our discussion begins with integrative medicine because it is foundational to the approaches described in this book. Integrative medicine brings evidence-informed complementary and conventional medicine together in a coordinated manner. This approach is a more recent development in health care, focusing on practices that promote psychological, mental, physical, and spiritual health for the whole family during all stages of treatment (NIH-NCCIH, 2021). In 2017, the Society for Integrative Oncology (SIO) formed a special interest group of international professionals in pediatric oncology to advance understanding of the field. The definition this group created to describe pediatric integrative oncology

DOI: 10.4324/9781003134800-1

underlies the principles discussed throughout this book: Pediatric integrative oncology] is

> a relationship-centered, evidence-informed, personalized approach to the whole child and family system utilizing mind and body practices, natural products and/or lifestyle modifications alongside conventional oncology care. Pediatric integrative oncology is offered throughout the illness trajectory to optimize health and wellness, enhance healing, minimize suffering, improve quality of life, and empower children and families to become active participants before, during, and beyond cancer treatment.
> (Tortora et al., 2021, p. 1)

The focus on whole person health – to improve and restore each individual's overall health rather than focusing solely on the disease and its symptoms – is especially important when working with a particularly vulnerable population: families with infants and young children who have complex medical conditions. How often do we hear the statement "Don't worry; babies are too young to remember and understand" in an attempt to soothe distraught parents during a difficult procedure? What if this is not true? What is the baby's emotional experience during repeated medical interventions, and what impact might this have on their development? How can we best support the emotional and social development of an infant or young child when there is an overwhelming, potentially life-threatening, medical condition that rightfully takes center stage?

Infant mental health research informs us that loving, secure relationships act as a stabilizing buffer during stressful encounters. But medical illness in early childhood affects the whole family. It is challenging for parents to maintain a healthy, loving relationship with their baby when confronted with such complex stresses as assisting in invasive medical procedures, understanding their baby may grow into a child with long-term difficulties, and the potential death of their baby (Melamed, 2010).

This book presents the application of DMT in pediatric medical settings to address these questions, focusing on how to approach the seemingly impossible juggle that is necessary to keep the baby's medical needs and emotional and felt experiences in mind, while also supporting parents through this life-changing journey. The foundational principles of pediatric medical DMT focus on the young child's embodied experiences and their manifestation in the child's behaviors and family dynamics, from the perspective of nonverbal interactional and relational experiences. DMT's focus on the body as an expressive tool for intervention uniquely addresses both the psychic and somatic aspects of the infant's experience of illness. Integral to this method is the use of nonverbal analysis to observe the qualitative elements of the infant's movement style to understand the baby's cues and preverbal experience.

DMT supports the infant/child's emotional life during the medical experience, taking into consideration subtle and more obvious effects on the child's later emotional and social development and other behaviors. DMT strives to establish a safe environment that enables the young child and family to share their emotional responses and manage difficult medical procedures, while creating and preserving loving, playful early childhood experiences and memories.

Infant mental health research reveals that babies do perceive their environment and remember adverse experiences (Gaensbauer, 1995, 2002, 2011). Early perception is registered through the baby's bodily felt experience, perceived through multisensory experiences, and informed by loving, secure interactions with primary caregivers (Gaensbauer, 2004). The "felt experience" refers to embodiment, which is a foundational concept used throughout this book. In brief, "embodiment" refers to the dynamic relationship that exists between perception, action, and emotion as experienced and expressed through unique, personal, nonverbal actions (Koch & Fischman, 2011; Sheets-Johnstone, 2011). It is only recently that more hospital programs are considering how the felt experience of having and being treated for an illness so early in life may affect the young child's current and future mental health (Kroupina & Elison, 2019; Lee et al., 2021; Zero to Three, 2016). The focus on embodiment is now a guiding principle used in DMT for intervention (Koch, 2006).

This notion of embodiment correlates to Stern's concept of body self (Stern, 1998), that is, in turn, very much related to the processes of self-development in the first years of life. Furthermore, parental embodiment is perceived by the infant and conveys vital cues to the parent's emotional stance, becoming a major component of the early parent–infant relationship. The quality of the parent–infant relationship and the family's emotional communication is at the core of mental health from infancy to adulthood (Sroufe et al., 2005). Pediatric life-threatening illness, a traumatic event for parents and infant, often derails the course of this growing relationship. Very young children "behave" their emotional distress rather than talk about it. So the role of child psychiatry at pediatric hospitals is to reflect with the parents on the link between their child's and their own behaviors during the traumatic event, articulating what the child and parents sense but often find unspeakable (Lieberman & Van Horn, 2008). Mothers who reported more difficulty in recognizing and understanding their child's mental states displayed decreased tolerance of distress on behavioral and self-report measures (Rutherford et al., 2015). Hence, facilitation of the parental reflective stance (Slade, 2005) to support increasing the awareness of parents and the psychiatry team of the infant's nonverbal communication is very much needed in these distressing medical situations. Adding the dance/movement therapy lens helps the caregivers and the whole medical team to read and understand the child's unique nonverbal communications. This empowers both the parent's and the child's senses of agency and control. The enjoyable activities in a dance/movement therapy session provide supportive ways to engage and strengthen their growing relationship, finding expression for these experiences that are difficult to articulate in words.

Goals of This Book

The idea for this book evolved out of years of dialogue between the authors, who both have specialties in infant mental health, to better support families and their children with medically complex conditions, and the medical teams that work so attentively with them, and to bring this knowledge to a wider audience. The lens of a child psychiatrist, Keren, provides a more thorough view into the family dynamics, including intervention strategies to support healthy development and prevent later emotional and behavioral disturbances. Collaborating with a dance/movement therapist who also has expertise in nonverbal communication analysis, Tortora, adds an in-depth awareness of the unspoken needs often expressed through subtle and overlooked cues. We share the belief that psychic and somatic processes are interwoven, and we have worked together for many years on the nonverbal aspects of communication between parents, infants, and therapists. The idea of focusing on how to alleviate the distress of very young children who are severely ill and to prevent the long-term sequelae of traumatic experiences on a child's mental health emerged from these years of collaboration. Further examples of our joint thinking are shared in the clinical discussions that follow the vignettes in each chapter.

This book also demonstrates how to build a treatment plan based on the infant or toddler's embodied experience, within the context of treating the whole family system during the medical experience (Tortora, 2019). The emotional and social strengths and weaknesses in each member of the family are considered within the context of the whole environment. This book fills a gap in the literature, for it introduces a pediatric treatment approach that – at its core – focuses on the very young pediatric patient's felt experience as it manifests in the child's behaviors and the family relational dynamics. By placing the primary focus on the messages our bodies speak, it gives voice to those aspects of the medical experience that have no words. This innovative approach to healing brings together a variety of fields, including infant mental health, infant and child psychiatry, nonverbal-movement analysis, somatic psychology, and the creative arts therapies. Evidence-based research from these professions is used to inform the clinical practices discussed in this book.

Our hope is that this book will stimulate much-needed future research, for there is a great sparsity of research in medical dance/movement therapy and no research specifically in pediatric dance/movement therapy with very young children (Bradt et al., 2015; Goodill, 2018). Vignettes from years during and after the medical experience presented throughout the text draw upon our work both in medical pediatric hospitals and private clinical practice, highlighting our unique perspectives and years of collaboration. In all vignettes, all names and identifying facts about the child, family members, and other social details have been changed to protect privacy. In some cases, the vignettes represent composites of sessions with different patients to provide further anonymity. In addition, use of gender pronouns is varied throughout to create gender neutrality. The vignettes also attempt to provide cultural, ethnic, and spiritual/religious diversity to promote understanding and respect for the unique psychosocial needs of all families.

Addressing Cultural Aspects of Medical Care

Culturally sensitive practice is currently a prominent focus in the larger context of the workplace and health care. A comprehensive discussion of this extensive topic goes beyond the focus of this book, in which we discuss some key components we consider when working with families. Cultural practices and spiritual beliefs form the basis of human behavior, and quality care requires that a medical team be both culturally sensitive and culturally competent (Wiener et al., 2013).

> The effect of cultural systems of values on health outcomes is huge, within and across cultures, in multicultural settings . . . the need to understand the relation between culture and health, especially the cultural factors that affect health-improving behaviors, is now crucial.
> (Napier et al., 2014, p. 1607)

In a comprehensive review of 72 articles (Gray et al., 2014), cultural factors were shown to influence illness representations, reaction to diagnosis, illness disclosure patterns, complementary and alternative medicine use, management of medical procedures, coping strategies, and end-of-life issues. Infants and toddlers with life-limiting and life-threatening illnesses deserve a cultural reappraisal of how a medical team offers both curative treatment and the best possible quality of life. Cultural competence includes the role of culture in decision-making, in spoken and unspoken language, in the parents' communication with the child about the illness, and the meanings they attribute to pain and suffering.

Although the search for the meaning of pain, severe illness, and suffering is a universal psychological/metaphysical phenomenon, it varies very much across cultures. The perception of physical pain and the meaning one gives to it also varies by culture (Davidhizar & Giger, 2004) and may impact the request for analgesic medications. Choice of treatment for children with critical illnesses may also be impacted by cultural differences. Specific coping strategies used by parents of children with cancer vary substantially by culture, too (Gray et al., 2014).

This mass of knowledge has several clinical implications (Wiener et al., 2013). Since family beliefs differ within a cultural community, to avoid stereotypes, one must initially assess a family's religious beliefs, rituals, and dietary practices, the parents' perception and fears regarding the illness, and their desired role in caring for their ill child. In relation to the reduction of the child's pain and distressing symptoms, one needs to assess the family attitudes and beliefs around pain and suffering. It is also essential not to impose mental health services because, in some cultures, emotional well-being is a private family issue. Understanding how the family defines and manages their child's cancer can guide the medical team in delivering holistic, culturally competent care (Thibodeaux & Deatrick, 2007).

Dance/Movement Therapy: A Bridge Between Nonverbal and Verbal Communication in Culturally Sensitive Practice

Deep communication is critical in situations where the child has a serious medical condition (Campbell, 2006). Mismatches in communication may lead to incorrect diagnosis, inadequate pain management, and/ or use of prescription medications and difficulty in obtaining parents' informed consent. Communication and language challenges influence the parents' role in caring for their child and make it difficult to learn complex medical terminology. Parents can despair, too, when language barriers prevent them from getting complete information about their child's medical status and prognosis. Parents may also miss out on services and resources (Gulati et al., 2012). The challenge is far beyond the task of mere translation, because the choice of words may impinge on successful communication.

The family of a child with a severe medical illness may not overtly express cultural barriers, and this can result in the misinterpretation of medical information and therapies. Beliefs and cultural practices vary with the diversity of education and Western acculturation, and families may feel obliged to conform to practices that differ greatly from their own beliefs, values, and practices. Facading, or the act of showing an outer appearance that may be misinterpreted by others, is a concept used in pediatric cancer to describe a latent pattern of behavior in transcultural-care interactions. Facading is important to consider (Pergert, 2017) for how it impacts familial responses. Medical teams need to be attuned to verbal and nonverbal messages the family conveys around issues of pain and illness, because good communication in pediatric cancer care means having a culturally informed clinical and research agenda.

Using a dance/movement therapeutic approach can be an extremely valuable asset to the medical team because it goes beyond verbal communication, using nonverbal analysis, music, and movement – all universal ways of expressing the whole array of our emotions – to support the child and family. In addition to the socioeconomic, educational, cultural, religious, and ethnic differences that are observed through spoken conversations, these differences and customs are also – and at times, more readily – revealed nonverbally. As exemplified in the vignettes throughout this book, the primary and thorough attention the dance/movement therapist pays to the nonverbal cues of all the family members enables the therapist to be sensitive to these important aspects of the family's needs (Tortora, 2019). We hope that this book supports the whole medical team by adding a deeper awareness of the value of nonverbal communication in providing culturally sensitive care.

Chapter Overview

Chapter 1 provides a literature review of the key infant mental health researchers and theorists who discuss the importance of bodily experience, highlighting the essential relational basis of bodily experience and movement as core ways preverbal children communicate. This chapter includes literature and research in infant mental health that address the baby's experiences occurring outside of conscious awareness. An important theme of this chapter distinguishes between the attachment relationship from the perspective of attachment theory and the nature and quality of the relationship specifically as it relates to parenting a baby with a medical illness.

Chapter 2 begins with an overview of how the term "embodiment" has been used to reflect the interrelatedness of the body and mind in the fields of psychology, cognitive science, neuroscience, linguistics, philosophy, affect neuroscience, somatics, and dance/movement therapy. This perception of embodiment takes into consideration the inevitably relational nature of bodily experience. An understanding of implicit and explicit memory within the context of embodiment, trauma treatment, and its clinical implications provides a deeper understanding of embodiment as it relates to the baby's bodily felt experience during medical treatment.

Chapter 3 explains how the concepts in Chapter 1 and Chapter 2 relate to the principles of pediatric medical dance/movement therapy. Medical dance/movement therapy is described as a body–mind–emotional psychotherapeutic approach for adults, children, and families, encouraging patients to express thoughts and feelings through movement, music, and verbal processing. This chapter elaborates on this definition through discussion and examples specifically related to the pediatric population. Included in this discussion is how dance therapists create an embodied holding environment by attending to body-to-body sensorially rich nonverbal dialogue that occurs among themselves, young patients, and caregivers. This dialogue occurs as the therapist simultaneously stays attuned to her own experience. Through this whole-body listening, the dance therapist focuses on the multisensory sensations, images, and feeling states that arise to analyze her own "embodied countertransference" reactions (Tortora, 2019, p. 10).

Chapter 4 discusses how an awareness of the young child's regulatory and multisensory processing can be used to support the child and the parent–child relationship. A vital aspect of building a secure attachment includes parents being able to accurately read their baby's arousal/behavioral states. The baby's shifting states of arousal, from deep sleep to awake to alert to distress, greatly affect the baby's ability to stay interested and engaged with her environment. In addition, the parents' ability to soothe their baby as the baby shifts from state to state greatly affects their sense of successful parenting. A review of research and literature that focuses on the role of regulation, first attained in early infancy by achieving a homeostatic state, is included.

This chapter also introduces Tortora's Embodied Parenting program (Tortora, 2015), which teaches parents how to attend to their baby's and their own nonverbal cues and integrates practices from different cultures using dance and music to soothe and engage babies, supporting their developing attachment relationship.

Chapter 5 addresses the baby's experience and memory of pain through a discussion about events that can expose the young child with medical complexities to develop traumatic reactions. There was a time in recent history when it was thought that babies did not remember pain or any preverbal experiences; however, more recent work in trauma and post-traumatic stress disorders (PTSD) has demonstrated that traumatic experiences – including early childhood traumatic events – are stored in lower parts of the brain and can be triggered by multisensory stimulations many years later (Perry & Pollard, 1998; Perry & Szalavitz, 2017; Perry & Winfrey, 2021; Porges & Daniel, 2017; Terr, 1992; van der Kolk, 2015). A thorough review of the literature and research focusing on trauma substantiates this focus. How these theories and research particularly relate to the baby's experience of her illness, treatment, pain, and memory development is also elucidated in this chapter.

Chapter 6 presents a concise history of the treatment experience of young pediatric patients in hospitals, including one-time hospital stays, extended stays, and repeated visits to the hospital. This chapter also discusses how hospitals and medical teams have historically tried to address the quality of life of the baby and the family; the importance of the presence of family members, and how and when this became a standard part of the hospital experience; and the history of pain management, including the absence of analgesics for infants. Also featured in this chapter is how the child life profession developed to support both the patient and the family.

Chapter 7 starts with a review of the long-term impact of life-threatening chronic illnesses, with emphasis on the embedded uncertainty and pain experience. Most of the longitudinal studies on the psychological impact of life-threatening illness in early childhood are about cancer, although uncertainty and pain are important factors that influence long-term psychological functioning regardless of the type of illness. This section is followed by a focus on the neurodevelopmental and psychological impacts of pediatric cancer on survivors, who frequently experience delayed and long-term effects of the disease and its intensive treatment, including chronic pain and other medical conditions, and cognitive, behavioral and emotional impairment. This chapter ends with clinical vignettes to illustrate how dance/movement therapy can be beneficial to the child and parents in the years after the acute phase of an illness.

Chapter 8 introduces the newly revised DC: 0–5™: *Diagnostic Classification of Mental Health and Developmental Disorders of Infancy and Early Childhood (DC: 0–5™)* (Zero to Three, 2016). This tool is structured in a multiaxial format reflecting: the child's symptoms clustered into clinical disorder categories (Axis I), the caregiving environment (Axis II), the child's physical health (Axis III), environmental psychosocial stressors (Axis IV), and the child's developmental strengths and weaknesses (Axis V). In this chapter, Keren shows how the use of this multiaxial formulation can be especially helpful in complex cases when physical and emotional aspects of the infant's development are at significant risk. A vignette from Tortora's private practice illustrates the clinical use of the *DC 0–5™*.

Chapter 9 provides an overview of select assessments and observation tools that include nonverbal measures to evaluate the young child's somatic and psychic distress. It ends with an assessment tool Tortora created, Dyadic Attachment-based Nonverbal Communicative Expressions (DANCE), derived from these assessments and Tortora's nonverbal analysis training. This chapter also highlights the specific nonverbal qualities she focuses on to understand the dynamics of the parent–child relationship in the treatment setting.

Chapter 10 provides an in-depth discussion about the use of rhythms, rocking, song, and dance to soothe and engage the young child and caregivers. The discussion includes how the field of music therapy uses rhythm and song with medical populations, as well as the role of dance, music, and rhythmic activities used around the world to both soothe and engage babies. Specific techniques that provide joyful ways for parents to play with their babies while learning how to attune to their unique styles of relating, which may be affected by their medical condition, are exemplified.

Chapter 11 introduces Multisensory Dance/Movement Psychotherapy (MSDMT), a specific pain management approach Tortora developed to help young children and their parents cope with medical procedures they experience as painful or scary. MSDMT is the application of DMT with an added emphasis on the role of the body and multisensory experience to support physiologic and psychological coping, specifically related to medical illness. It is a noninvasive method that complements pharmacological/ medical treatments. Tortora (2019, p. 4) refers to MSDMT as an "embodied analgesic" that supports the patient to attune to somato-sensorial sensation to engage and soothe by creating a sense empowerment and coping. MSDMT treatment includes supporting the attachment relationships by incorporating the whole family during treatment. A discussion of this technique is exemplified with case vignettes.

Chapter 12 is a synthesis of the all the information in this book in outline form. It provides the professional with the key concepts of dance/ movement therapy, child psychiatry, and infant mental health to best support parents and family members coping with having a young child with a medical condition.

Appendices provide detailed examples of dance/movement therapy–based practices to best support the child and their caregivers, augmenting the concepts in this book. "My Body Speaks! Getting to Know Me in the Hospital" is a printable handout that parents and caregivers can fill out to help the medical team understand their child's specific nonverbal styles of communication and engaging.

Conclusion

When an infant or young child's life is threatened by medical illness, it is crucial that the medical professionals and family keep their focus on saving the child's life as well as supporting the child and family's emotional experience. As discussed throughout this book, receiving a diagnosis of a serious medical condition with a baby or young child takes a profound emotional toll on the patient and the whole family. During this time, attention to the body–mind–biopsychosocial experience of the young child may not always be the main focus. The high-intensity and long-term treatment protocols of some pediatric illnesses impact the quality of life of the whole family system.

The influence of the caregiver-infant relationship encompasses both the parents and the medical team, first introduced as the "Cancer – WWW" perspective (Tortora, 2019, p. 7) but revised to "Pediatric – WWW" perspective to encompass all pediatric illnesses. In this view, caring for a young child with a medical illness must involve looking at the Whole child; taking into consideration the Whole family system experience; and working in collaboration with the Whole medical team to build a sense of community. Using the word "whole" upholds the awareness of the embodied experience for each participant, to preserve the quality of life for the child and family throughout the medical treatment continuum. The use of whole also supports the DMT and integrative medicine perspective of empowering family members and the patient to actively participate in their medical care (Tortora, 2019; Witt, 2017).

The goal of this book is to introduce pediatric medical DMT in the context of infant mental health and child psychiatry and to reach a wider audience. We hope to demonstrate that DMT is an underutilized specialty that can contribute a great deal to support young children with medical illnesses and their families. Grounded in a biopsychosocial perspective, the inherently nonverbal and embodied nature of pediatric medical DMT is exceptionally well-positioned as a strong component of integrative medicine services.

References

Bradt, J., Shim, M., & Goodill, S. W. (2015, January 7). Dance/movement therapy for improving psychological and physical outcomes in cancer patients. *Cochrane Database of Systematic Reviews, 1*, CD007103. https://doi.org/10.1002/14651858.CD007103.pub3

Campbell, A. (2006). Spiritual care for sick children of five world faiths. *Paediatric Nursing, 18*, 22–25.

Davidhizar, R., & Giger, J. (2004). A review of the literature on care of clients in pain who are culturally diverse. *International Nursing Review, 51*, 47–55.

Gaensbauer, T. (1995). Trauma in the preverbal period. Symptoms, memories, and developmental impact. *Psychoanal Study Child, 50*, 122–149. https://doi.org/10.1080/00797 308.1995.11822399

Gaensbauer, T. (2002). Representations of trauma in infancy: Clinical and theoretical implications for the understanding of early memory. *Infant Mental Health Journal, 23*(3), 259–277.

Gaensbauer, T. (2004). Telling their stories: Representation and reenactment of traumatic experiences occurring in the first year of life. *Zero to Three, 24*(5), 25–31.

Gaensbauer, T. (2011). Embodied simulation, mirror neurons, and reenactment of trauma in early childhood. *Neuropsychoanalysis, 13*(1), 91–107.

Goodill, S. (2018). Accumulating evidence for dance/movement therapy in cancer care. *Frontiers in Psychology, 9*(1778). https://doi.org/10.3389/fpsyg.2018.01778

Gray, W., Szulczewski, L., Regan, S., Williams, J., & Ahna, P. (2014). Cultural influences in pediatric cancer: From diagnosis to cure/end of life. *Journal of Pediatric Oncology Nursing, 31*, 252–271.

Gulati, S., Watt, L., Shaw, N., Sung, L., Poureslami, I., Klaassen, R., Dix, D., & Klassen, A. (2012). Communication and language challenges experienced by Chinese and South Asian immigrant parents of children with cancer in Canada: Implications for health services delivery. *Pediatric Blood Cancer, 58*, 572–578.

Koch, S. (2006). Interdisciplinary embodiment approaches. Implications for creative arts therapies. In S. K. I. Bräuninger (Ed.), *Advances in dance/movement therapy. Theoretical perspectives and empirical findings* (pp. 17–28). Logos.

Koch, S., & Fischman, D. (2011). Embodied enactive dance/movement therapy. *American Journal of Dance Therapy, 33*, 57–32.

Kroupina, M., & Elison, K. (2019, July). The pediatric birth to three clinic and early childhood mental health program, meeting the needs of complex pediatric patients. *Zero to Three*, 31–34.

Lee, D., Serrano, V., von Schulz, J., Fields, D., & Buchholz, M. (2021). From patients to partners: Promoting health equity in pediatric primary care with the HealthySteps program. *Zero to Three, 42*(2), 72–78.

Lieberman, A., & Van Horn, P. (2008). *Psychotherapy with infants and young children: Reparing the effects of stress and trauma on early attachment.* The Guilford Press.

Melamed, B. G. (2010). Parenting the chronically ill infant. In S. Tyano, M. Keren, H. Hermann, & J. Cox (Eds.), *Parenthood and mental health. A bridge between inafnt and adult psychiatry* (pp. 277–288.). Wiley Blackwell.

Napier, A., Ancarno, C., Butler, B., et al. (2014). Culture and health. *Lancet, 384*, 1607–1639.

NIH-NCCIH. (2021). *Complementary, alternative, or integrative health: What's in a name?* Retrieved June 30, 2021 from www.nccih.nih.gov/health/complementary-alternative-or-integrative-health-whats-in-a-name

Pergert, P. (2017). Facading in transcultural interactions: Examples from pediatric cancer care in Sweden. *Psycho Oncology, 26*, 1013–1018.

Perry, B., & Pollard, R. (1998). Homeostasis, stress, trauma, and adaptation. A neurodevelopmental view of childhood trauma. *Child & Adolescent Psychiatry Clinics of North America., 7*, 33–51.

Perry, B., & Szalavitz, M. (2017). *The boy who was raised as a dog: What traumatized children can teach us about loss, love and healing* (3rd ed.). Basic Books.

Perry, B., & Winfrey, O. (2021). *What happened to you? Conversations on trauma, resilience, and healing.* Flatiron Books.

Porges, S. W., & Daniel, S. (2017). Play and dynamics of treating pediatric medical trauma. In S. Daniel & C. Trevarthen (Eds.), *Rhythms of relating in children's therapies: Connecting creatively with vunerable children* (pp. 113–124). Jessica Kingsley Publishers.

Rutherford, H. J., Booth, C. R., Luyten, P., Bridgett, D. J., & Mayes, L. C. (2015, August). Investigating the association between parental reflective functioning and distress tolerance in motherhood. *Infant Behavior and Development, 40*, 54–63. https://doi.org/10.1016/j.infbeh.2015.04.005

Sheets-Johnstone, M. (2011). *The primacy of movement* (2nd ed.). John Benjamin's Publishing Company.

Slade, A. (2005, September). Parental reflective functioning: An introduction. *Attachment & Human Development, 7*(3), 269–281. https://doi.org/10.1080/14616730500245906

Sroufe, L., Egeland, B., Carlson, E., & Collins, W. (2005). *The development of the person: The Minnesota study of risk and adaptation from birth to adulthood.* The Guilford Press.

Stern, D. (1998). *The interpersonal world of the infant: A view from psychoanalysis and developmental psychology.* Taylor & Francis Ltd.

Terr, L. (1992). *Too scared to cry: How trauma affects children . . . and untimately us all.* Basic Books.

Thibodeaux, A., & Deatrick, J. (2007). Cultural influence on family management of children with cancer. *Journal of Pediatric Oncology Nursing, 24*, 227–233.

Tortora, S. (2015). The importance of being seen – Winnicott, dance movement psychotherapy and the embodied experience. In M. Spelman & F. Thomson-Salo (Eds.), *The Winnicott tradition: Lines of development – evolution of theory and practice over the decades.* Karnac.

Tortora, S. (2019). Children are born to dance! Pediatric medical dance/movement therapy: The view from integrative pediatric oncology. *Children, 6*(14), 1–27. https://doi.org/10.3390/children6010014

Tortora, S., Raghunathan, N. J., Seifert, G., Sibinga, E. M. S., & Ghelman, R. (2021, March 1). A comprehensive definition for pediatric integrative oncology through an

international consensus. *Complementary Therapies in Medicine, 57*, 102678. https://doi.org/
https://doi.org/10.1016/j.ctim.2021.102678

van der Kolk, B. (2015). *The body keeps the score: Brain, mind and body in the healing of trauma.*
Penguin Books.

Wiener, L., McConnell, D., Latella, L., & Ludi, E. (2013). Cultural and religious consider-
ations in pediatric palliative care. *Palliat Support Care, 11*, 47–67.

Witt, C., Balneaves, L., Cardoso, M., Cohen, L., Greenlee, H., Johnstone, P., Kucuk, O.,
Mailman, J., & Mao, J. (2017). A comprehensive definition for integrative oncology.
Journal of the National Cancer Institute Monographs, 52, 3–8.

Zero to Three. (2016). *Diagnostic classification of mental health and developmental disorders of
infancy and early childhood: DC: 0–5.* Zero To Three Press.

Chapter 1

The Role of the Baby's Body, Nonverbal-Movement Experience, and Communication in Building the Caregiver-Baby Relationship

Introduction

Parents who are attuned and responsive to their baby's nonverbal actions enable the baby to feel his actions are communicative and have been seen and heard. Winnicott, a British pediatrician and psychoanalyst who was especially significant in establishing developmental psychology and object relations theory, highlights the parents' role in his simple statement: "When I look I am seen, so I exist" (1982, p. 16). From the infant's point of view, this quote describes the experience of engaging with a nurturing mother figure. It also acknowledges how a baby comes to gain a sense of herself through early action-based experiences with primary caregivers. The act of looking, which requires a physical motion, informs the baby's emotional and social formation of self. Through this emotionally rich, bodily felt exchange, the baby understands that she matters, and this is at the heart of building a healthy sense of self in relationship to others.

The capacity for attunement requires emotional availability on the part of the caregiver/parent. Any very stressful situation, such as a serious pediatric illness, may compromise the parents' availability and unconsciously undermine the infant's sense of self. This chapter explains the significant role the felt, bodily experience plays in psychological development, focusing on how the young child's psyche – body, mind, soul, and spirit – develops within the context of a newly forming parent–child relationship and how it may be affected by complex medical experiences.

Throughout this book, early research on the mother figure is presented to accurately describe how these theories and findings relate to the pediatric patient's experience, while taking into consideration the important role all significant caregivers play in a young child's life. The word "mother" will be used when referencing classic research, specifically with mothers and babies; the terms "mother figure," "parents," "caregiver," and "significant caregivers" will be used interchangeably to be inclusive of other meaningful relationships in the baby's world, which can be especially important in the early life of a baby with a medical illness.

DOI: 10.4324/9781003134800-2

The Baby's Bodily Experience Within the Context of Relationships

For babies, the earliest positive experiences of themselves occur through their bodily actions, communications, and sensations within the context of supportive relationships. Stern, an infant psychiatrist whose work has also been influential in our understanding of emotional development in babies, takes Winnicott's concepts further, stating: "Infants are not 'lost at sea' in a wash of abstractable qualities of experience"; instead, they use these physically felt interactions to identify and differentiate self from other, gradually and systematically organizing their sense of self, operating "out of awareness as the experiential matrix from which thought and perceived forms and identifiable acts and verbalized feeling will later arise" (1985, p. 67). Stern attributes to the baby an earlier agency over his sense of self by acknowledging that the baby engages in relational experiences from pre-existing corporeal sensations that create a sense of agency and physical cohesion, which the baby uses to build concepts of self that are distinct from other. Stern places the infant's sense of self – which develops prior to self-awareness – as the central and primary organizing reference point from which interpersonal development and social functioning occur (Stern, 1985, p. 6).

Winnicott and Stern both emphasize that the baby's psyche-soma connection develops through the baby's early bodily felt experiences that occur within meaningful relationships. This psyche-soma experience of self with others is the basis for the formation of the mind, distinct from the psyche, and includes a symbolic sense of self. In Stern's definition, sense of self draws attention to direct experiences that create patterns of awareness derived from actions and mental activities. His term "core self" describes the experiential sense of self that occurs outside of conscious awareness, related to sensations, affects, actions, and time spent with the baby's own being (Stern, 1985). The felt and proprioceptive feedback of self-actions provide self-coherence, informing the infant's awareness of self, differentiated from other. Winnicott uses the term "indwelling" (1960, p. 590) to explain the infant's positive integration of the psyche-soma experience of her own body, mind, and psyche. Indwelling describes the infant's development of her psychic self, emerging from the experience of her own body, evolving from the infant's motor, sensory, and functional experiences, creating a separate "me" from others: "not-me." Through indwelling, the baby forms a body scheme. These traditional developmental psychology and psychoanalytic theories reference body experiences in the early psychic and psychosocial stages, with an emphasis on their role in more complex cognitive modes of processing, self-awareness, and identity.

Tortora's "sense of body" concept extends these theories to place primary emphasis on bodily experience as a central source in the development of self, which lives and is maintained in the body and is expressed through nonverbal communication. This additional way of viewing bodily experiences is very important to consider when working with young children who have medical conditions that greatly impact their bodily felt experiences during this significant stage in the development of self-concepts.

Sense of Body Concept and Clinical Implications

Trained as a dance/movement psychotherapist, Tortora builds upon the ideas of Winnicott and Stern, putting greater emphasis on the multisensory-nonverbal-embodied experience as primary and present throughout life, without always being translated into a consciously directed or conceptually thought self. Tortora's (2006, p. 31) sense of body concept postulates that the baby's early body-based experiences shape how the baby communicates, explores, and organizes intrapersonal and interpersonal experiences. Tortora (2006, 2015) differentiates sense of body from sense of self, putting more emphasis on embodied experiences. These experiences can be fueled by intersubjective motivation, influencing how the baby gets to know and express self on all developmental levels. Sense of body in contrast to the core self-concept goes beyond a perceptual-cognitive process of a symbolic representation of self, viewing the embodied felt experience as primary and all-encompassing throughout development. It focuses on how nonverbal experiences – including touch, motion, gesture, posture, and proprioceptive and interoceptive sensations – occur in response to and during social relationships, influencing the baby's developing understanding of self. Affect, cognition, and the emotional expressivity of communication are infused by these body-based multisensory felt sensations. Physical actions, as small as a breath or as large as a leg kick, involve sensations that confirm an infant's agency. Self-initiated actions create a sense of "I do." The kinesthetic and environmental feedback from the action creates a sense of "I am able." Actions and physical sensations that have significance or are repeated become, over time, nonverbal patterns that are codified into the child's personal movement signature. "I am able" becomes "I am." Fundamentally, the baby's sense of body is how she experiences and gets to know self, and from which a sense of self on emotional, cognitive, symbolic, social, spiritual, and communicative levels emerges. Caldwell (2016, p. 226), a dance therapist who references somatic approaches in her DMT theoretical and clinical model, aptly discusses the role of the body in the formation of identity to describe body identity development:

> It may be that cognition itself, previously held as a solely mental phenomenon that constructs and elaborates identity, can be re-positioned as a central somatic event. Instead of *I think, therefore I am*, perhaps we can state *I move (and sense), therefore I think* (emphasis in original).

In applying these concepts to the clinical pediatric situation, we may ask: How does a baby's medical illness inform and affect the experience of his body in the formulation of self? How does the baby incorporate sensations that at the very least inhibit smooth bodily functioning and movement exploration, and at the very worst create felt perceptions that are painful and potentially life threatening? How does the intrusion of medically necessary procedures, performed outside of the baby's exploratory and willful actions, contribute to the maturing psychological, cognitive, and sensational self? How does the infant's exposure to bright lights, noxious odors, loud and uncomfortable auditory stimuli, temperature fluctuations, abrasive tactile sensations, and more inform his psyche-soma experience?

> Angel, an 11-month-old baby with severe combined immunodeficiency disease (SCID), is a new patient at the hospital. Though he has only recently been admitted, within his first three days, he is frequently left without any family members during the entire day, as his father works long hours and his mother has three other children at home. Angel is a relatively strong, curious baby who has taken to pulling out his intravenous lines. Three nurses enter to place a new line. Upon their entry, Angel, who had been lying in his crib, a bit sleepy, suddenly sits up, his eyes darting back and forth as he scans the faces of each adult. He scampers to the corner of his crib, appearing alert and vigilant. The nurses approach with a kindness that belies the task at hand. Having experienced Angel's ability to resist such procedures, they are also concerned about how to proceed with their next steps. As anticipated, Angel begins to flail his body, kick his legs, and swing his arms. The atmosphere in the room becomes tense as the nurses silently circle the crib, thinking through how to safely proceed. Angel's eyes dash around the room without pause. I wonder whether he is attempting to find a safe, warm gaze to hold him through his obvious distress. I visually attempt to enter his field of view, but given his frantic, arrhythmic darting, he does not see me. Simultaneously, he flicks his tongue to and fro in his mouth, shrieking. In my empathic reflection, I sense that he may feel his eyes, tongue, and voice are the only parts of himself over which he has sole control. The nurses do not want to stoke Angel's fears, so they don't proceed, and decide to try to accomplish their task again later. All are noticeably shaken.

Clinical Discussion

From these behaviors, it is clear that Angel has endured medical procedures that require his body to be restrained against his will. This can be necessary during infant medical procedures, and how these experiences get imprinted in the baby's body is an important consideration.

On one hand, parents are commonly told that the children are so young they will not remember their experiences during difficult procedures. On the other hand, recent trauma research acknowledges that preverbal experiences do manifest in the body and remain present through memories that are held in the body (Cloitre et al., 2009; van der Kolk, 2015). The term "held in the body" refers to gestures, postures, sensations, and numbness or pain located anywhere in the body that are detached from the memory and not associated with the trauma, but are related to the traumatic experience(s). Winnicott (1972, p. 16) states, "The self finds itself naturally placed in the body but may, in certain circumstances, become dissociated from the body or the body from it." The use of the word "dissociated" is important in this statement because it implies that the felt experience may become separated from conscious thought and memory. This can be healthy and help to build resilience; however, it may also remain in the body as a traumatic embodied memory, manifesting as problematic behaviors that may not be understood as being associated with the early traumatic experiences. Working from the perspective that the young patient's sense of self is present from birth, and that he gains knowledge about himself and his world through his sense of body, these medical experiences must contribute to his developing relationship with and experience of his body, mind, and psyche.

As a child psychiatrist, Keren is often asked whether an 11-month-old baby will remember such a negative experience. We know that he will. There is quite a lot of research about implicit preverbal memory and post-traumatic symptoms in the first years of life. Angel's vigilant attitude, observed as soon as the nurses enter his room, is actually a behavioral enactment of his memory of previous experiences with nurses; the nurses are concrete reminders of his pain.

From Tortora's description of the case, Angel has become increasingly vigilant when any member of the hospital team enters his room and may be looking for a protective attachment figure. To break his association with the idea that anyone entering his room will hurt him, Tortora adapts a very gentle approach when entering his room in subsequent sessions:

> Now I start each session by speaking to him kindly from the door, alerting him that I am here to play. I wait for him to look toward my voice, and I smile when he does. If he averts his eyes, I wait, singing a hello song to him in a calm, slow melody, matching the rhythm of his breath pattern.

In Tortora's subsequent and consistent very gentle approach, she uses reassuring words and singing in an attempt to act as a replacement attachment figure. Current research shows that the close proximity of a main attachment figure during an adverse event is one of the strongest protective factors against post-traumatic stress disorder (PTSD) in infants and young children (Kroupina & Elison, 2019). We must impress upon parents the importance of their presence, with an understanding of the real-life struggles they face, and without making them feel guilty. In the absence of a main attachment figure from the family, it is helpful to choose a member or a few members of the hospital team, such as the dance therapist, other integrative medicine practitioners, nursing support staff, or a child-life specialist, who can develop an attachment relationship with the young child and be present to provide comfort during procedures that the child perceives as stressful or painful. Also, the infant needs to be told explicitly that when his parents are not with him, they do not forget him, that they love him very much, and they know how much he would like to keep them close during the painful treatments he fears. Keeping a photograph of his close family members can help, too.

Tortora makes this suggestion during the next session she has with Angel when his father is present. She first emphasizes how excited Angel is to have his father at the hospital, specifically pointing to his actions – bouncing up and down as he reaches to him – that provide nonverbal cues. Tortora expresses her understanding that Dad can't always be present when Angel is getting treatment. She asks Dad if he can leave behind a photograph of him and Angel's mother so Angel can look at it, stating, "This can help Angel keep you in his mind. Even though he is so young, he does have feelings and knows you are his family." These steps effectively support Angel and enable him to become more comfortable during his hospitalization. Dad demonstrates his understanding, for the next time Tortora has a session with Angel, there are photos in his crib of Dad, Mom, and siblings.

> Starting each session with Angel by pausing to sing the same hello song from the doorway, while attuning to his breath pattern, becomes our opening ritual. Angel now registers that our activities are interactive and playful. His vigilant stance is gone. When I enter, he pulls himself up, sitting in his crib. He orients his whole body toward me, watching me with an excited expression as I approach. Now he allows me to hold him as we dance around the room to bouncy beats or soothing lullabies, while we hold the photos of his parents.

Intersubjectivity and Communicative Musicality

Babies are social beings who are aware of and connect with their primary caregivers right from birth. Infants are born with mental structures that intrinsically link perceptions and actions, motivating them to seek social and emotional engagement by coordinating, matching, and complementing the psychological feeling states and tones of their significant caregivers (Trevarthen, 1980, 1998). Described by Trevarthen (1980, p. 316) as "intersubjectivity," this ability to engage in communicative give-and-take interactions creates a shared framework of meaning that emotionally connects the infant to the caregiver, a concept that has been well researched in the field of infant mental health (Stern, 1985). Intersubjectivity creates a joint social consciousness and identification that can be considered at the root of empathy.

In his early research, Trevarthen (1980) notes that by six weeks, the infant and caregiver's loving and joyful exchanges create a shared body state through rhythmic, dance-like movements and vocal patterns of engagement. The co-created melodic, rhythmic, and imitative vocal and nonverbal turn-taking interactions promote emotional regulation for both parent and baby. Trevarthen states that this musical dialogue satisfies our instinctive need for intimate companionship.

Trevarthen's student, Malloch, studied this rhythmic dance more deeply, realizing that there are inherent, measurable attributes to this motivated movement related to the pulse, quality, and narratives that occur during this exchange (Malloch, 2017). These qualities are elaborated on in Chapter 10, in the discussion about the use of rhythm for therapeutic intervention, and exemplified in the following vignette detailing a subsequent session with Angel and his mom. Central to this concept, called "communicative musicality" by Malloch and Trevarthen (2009, p. 4), is an emphasis on the sensitive, attuned, interactive sympatico of mother and baby, recognized as an innate human ability expressed through the nonverbal expressions of the infant and caregiver. The elements of dance/movement therapy for parents and young children naturally build on this inborn capability. Dance therapy not only helps the child; it can also be very helpful to parents as it highlights their important role and guides them in ways to engage their child, as illustrated by the following dance therapy session:

> Today when I enter, Dad and Mom are in the room, too, sitting in chairs next to Angel's crib. I greet them warmly, sharing how much Angel is enjoying looking at their photos during our dancing. They appear surprised yet pleased. I ask Mom what her favorite music is, and will she join our dancing, Looking at Angel, I exclaim, "Today, Angel, you can dance with Mom and Dad, in their arms!" We put on Mom's favorite salsa beat, and Angel immediately starts to rock up and down, matching the rhythm. He seems to know this rhythm deeply. Mom shares that it is always playing in their home, and she too becomes more animated. As she lifts Angel from his crib, he pulses his dangling legs to match the beat, and then firmly wraps them around her torso. They fall into such synchrony it is difficult to tell who is leading whom. Dad joins in and together we all dance around the room. Dad and Mom take turns holding and dancing with Angel. As we move through the space, at times I go toward them, lifting my

hands up to give Angel a high five, a gesture he is just beginning to master through our clapping dance-games.

Communicative musicality involves parents' and baby's sensitive attunement to the unspoken dynamic of the other's actions. Though this is a dynamic dyadic exchange, it is not an equal exchange. It is the primary caregiver's initial ability to read and attune to the baby's nonverbal cues that will impact the baby's sense of feeling seen. Ainsworth's (Ainsworth et al., 1978) research was the first to demonstrate that the quality of the mother figure's response to her baby's cues is a key factor that reflects the infant's later development of attachment security. To foster a secure attachment, the most central maternal organizing behavior identified in Ainsworth's research is "maternal sensitivity," defined as the mother's ability to perceive and interpret the baby's cues with accuracy, appropriateness, and promptness. Key to this sensitivity is the mother adjusting to baby's timing rather than directing the engagement. The qualities that create contingent responsiveness include the parent modifying specific nonverbal aspects of their actions and speech, such as decelerating, exaggerating, varying, and simplifying their engagement style to complement the baby's style (Papoušek, 2011). Successfully reading the baby's cues supports the growing secure relationship by creating ongoing moments of positive sequential reciprocal interactions, described by Papoušek as "angel's circles" (2011, p. 36). These attuned everyday preverbal communications build the infant's individual regulatory capacity. This successful dialogue constructs mutual co-regulation.

The lack of being held, emotionally and literally, by a parent due to a young child's medical fragility can disrupt development of a solid, reliable "continuity of being" in the Winnicottian sense. As discussed earlier, the baby learns about himself through the experience of being in his body, as well as through self and other explorations. When innate embodied explorations are limited due to restrictive medical apparatus that restrains movement explorations and comfortable body-to-body physical contact, we must consider how these conditions affect the infant's experiences of self and body scheme and the impact on the development of meaningful relationships. Drawing from the sense of body concept, which says that some experiences stay held within the body, the young pediatric patient's experience of her psyche-soma may be colored by a series of difficult sensations that have not been mitigated by the loving embrace of caregivers. These experiences are not translated through the conscious mind but held in the body of the baby and parents. When working with caregivers and their babies with medical illness, it behooves us to keep this understanding in mind. For some parents, especially those with poor coping mechanisms, past traumatic experiences and/or losses, and/or their own sickness, handling the stresses of their child's serious illness may be overwhelming.

Our task, as mental health professionals, is to detect these struggles early on during hospitalization to provide parents with intensive, sensitive, therapeutic support. We strive to develop activities that preserve the developing parent–infant relationship and the baby's psyche-soma experience.

Creating a Balance Between Exploratory and Proximity-Seeking Aspects of the Attachment System During the Medical Experience

A core component within the parent–infant attachment is the way the infant represents his caregiver's protective behavior in times of distress. Reading cues in general, and especially during distress, is considered a significant feature in creating a secure attachment. Bowlby (1969/1982) theorized that babies are biologically disposed to look for an attachment figure when they are in distress, and once established, freely explore their environment from this secure base, also described as a "safe haven." Optimally, these exploratory and proximity-seeking systems are in a balanced interplay; whenever the child is in distress, the attachment system is activated and the exploratory one is deactivated. A secure base, or safe haven, is the key ingredient in the relationships that provide emotional and physiological regulation and has been linked to the later development of empathy and mentalization skills. But parents vary in ability to provide protection and comfort in times of perceived danger. Bowlby stresses the existence of the attachment and exploration systems across age range, meaning severe distress in the parent will activate the parental-attachment system in parallel with the infant's system activation. This is especially relevant in extremely stressful situations when an infant is diagnosed with a serious and/or potentially life-threatening condition.

In adverse situations, the outcome for the child is the result of a complex interplay between risk and protective factors in the infant, caregivers, and their environment. While the parent's own attachment system is activated by these extremely stressful situations, it is important to note that a secure attachment is a protective factor for both the parent and infant coping with illness-related stresses. Sameroff and MacKenzie (2003) conceptualized the transactional epigenetic model to explain the variability of normal and abnormal developmental outcomes of children. Belsky and Fearon (2002) added complexity to this model by introducing the notion of a differential susceptibility to positive and negative life events based on the level of brain plasticity each individual was born with. These understandings make it quite difficult, if not impossible, to predict which parents and infants will grow or collapse from the tremendously stressful period. At one end of the spectrum, the infant may develop a need for self-reliance that can grow into strength and independence. Alternatively, it can foster deep-rooted fears or feelings of abandonment and, as Winnicott states, annihilation. The infant's own characteristics impact very much how he reacts to the illness. The parents' ability to provide a strong, consistent, safe, holding environment throughout the medical experience can boost their sense of successful parenting; however, the emotional pain, strife, and stress of not being able to protect their baby from illness and ensuing treatments can greatly impact the parents' confidence in their relationship with their child. For example, some parents react by withdrawing; others become intrusive. These parental behaviors then increase the infant's distress, which can result in difficulties parenting the child, creating a vicious circle of mutually negative feedback loops.

It is important to emphasize that this is not by any means placing blame or fault on the care by the parents or medical team; rather, it is an attempt to bring awareness to the complex conditions medical treatment may inadvertently create in the formation of self and the parent–child relationship. The medical experience deeply affects the whole family and leaves lasting impressions that can later surface in attitudes and behaviors that may at first appear unrelated to the early medical experience. For example, the child may become overly agitated when not feeling in control of her environment, quick to have a tantrum, and avoidant of touch – even when a parent provides loving touch. Parents may be overly protective or fearful of setting limits with the child, behaviors unconsciously informed by worry over upsetting their child.

The infant's temperament is a very important variable, as Woodhouse and colleagues (2019) have shown in their study of maternal responses to their temperamentally irritable babies (Cassidy et al., 2005). This research studied the mother's availability to soothe the baby during times of distress, when crying not fussing, through chest-to-chest holding until the infant was completely calm, picking up the infant after he strongly signaled this desire, and not presenting frightening responses to the infant. According to their findings, behaviors that promote a calm regulatory state during infant explorations include the ability to support calm connectedness; the ability to repair moments that interrupt the infant's ability to stay calmly regulated without terminating exploration; being available for eye contact when the infant is seeking social connection, while not soliciting eye contact that usurps the infant's capacity to set the pace; and sharing in delight when initiated by the infant. These behaviors demonstrate the caregiver's ability to read and anticipate the baby's cues and prevent stress and dysregulation when the baby is susceptible to distress. During these caregiving behaviors, the infant learns she can trust her parent to provide a safe, secure base.

Enabling parents of babies with a medical illness to use these specific nonverbal caregiver behaviors during distress, especially throughout and after medical care, has the potential to ease the baby's and parents' experience and support the caregiver-baby relationship. Including DMT activities that enable the young child to express her sensory-felt medical experience through movement, dance, music, and play can beneficially alter the baby's sense of body experience.

Conclusion

Starting from birth, it is through interactions that an individual builds their concept of self and self as distinct from other. Continuous and recurring patterns, created through interactive dynamics among the brain, body, and the environment, become embodied in memory and inform the infant's budding sense of self and reality. All infants first express their feelings, learn about the world, and develop their internal representations of self through their actions and behaviors upon the world around them. Focusing on the baby's experience of her body naturally directs us to the baby's significant relationships, because the infant's felt experiences inform how she develops social relationships.

This begins with the infant's primary significant caregivers, since all babies are dependent on the care of others to grow. Interpersonal experiences significantly shape how the baby comes to understand and perceive her selfhood. Keeping the baby's felt experience in the forefront is essential when working with very sick babies. As illustrated in the vignettes, using dance/movement therapy techniques provide a body-to-body avenue that both reflects and expresses the baby's and the parents' adverse experiences. This builds on the intersubjective nature of the parent-baby relationship through activities that intrinsically stimulate communicative musicality. The caregiver's ability to accurately read and respond to the baby's nonverbal cues can be instrumental in creating an embodied sense of safety that supports the attachment–exploration continuum, even within the context of the difficult medical experience. These behaviors include providing a calm, regulated presence during treatment and soothing the crying baby by holding her until she reaches a calm state after the treatment.

It is through these attuned experiences that we can preserve and nurture the communicative musicality experiences innate in the primary caregiver–infant relationship, building the baby's psyche, body, mind, soul, and spirit.

References

Ainsworth, M., Blehar, M., Waters, E., & Wall, S. (1978). *Patterns of attachment: A psychological study of the strange situation*. Erlbaum.

Belsky, J., & Fearon, R. (2002). Infant-mother attachment security, contextual risk, and early development: A moderational analysis. *Development & Psychopathology*, *14*, 293–310.

Bowlby, J. (1969/1982). *Attachment and loss: Attachment* (2nd ed., Vol. I). Basic Books.

Caldwell, C. (2016). Body identity development: Definitions and discussions. *Body, Movement and Dance in Psychotherapy*, *11*(4), 220–234. https://doi.org/10.1080/17432979.1145141

Cassidy, J., Woodhouse, S. S., Cooper, G., Hoffman, K., Powell, B., & Rodenberg, M. (2005). Examination of the precursors of infant attachment security: Implications for early intervention and intervention research. In Y. Z. L. J. Berlin, L. Amaya-Jackson, & M. T. Greenberg (Eds.), *Enhancing early attachments: Theory, research, intervention, and policy* (pp. 34–60). Guilford.

Cloitre, M., Stolbach, B., Herman, J., van de Kolk, B., Pynoos, R., Want, J., & Petkova, E. (2009). A developmental approach to complex PTSD: Childhood and adult cumulative trauma as predictors of symptom complexity. *Journal of Traumatic Stress, 22*(5), 399–408.

Kroupina, M., & Elison, K. (2019, July). The pediatric birth to three clinic and early childhood mental health program, meeting the needs of complex pediatric patients. *Zero to Three,* 31–34.

Malloch, S. (2017). Establishing a therapy of musicality: The embodied narrative of myself and others. In S. T. Daniel (Ed.), *Rhythms of relating in children's therapies: Connecting creatively with vulnerable children* (pp. 63–81). Jessica Kingsley Publishers.

Malloch, S., & Trevarthen, C. (2009). *Communicative musicality: Exploring the basis of human companionship.* Oxford University Press.

Papoušek, M. (2011). Resilience, strengths, and regulatory capacities: Hidden resources in developmental disorders of infant mental health. *Infant Mental Health Journal, 32*(1), 29–46.

Sameroff, A. J., & MacKenzie, M. J. (2003). Capturing transactional models of development: The limits of the possible. *Development & Psychopathology, 15,* 613–640.

Stern, D. (1985). *The interpersonal world of the infant.* Basic Books, Inc.

Tortora, S. (2006). *The dancing dialogue: Using the communicative power of movement with young children.* Paul H. Brookes Publishing Company.

Tortora, S. (2015). Dance/movement psychotherapy in early childhood treatment and pediatric oncology. In S. Chaiklin & H. Wengrower (Eds.), *The art and science of dance/movement therapy: Life is dance.* Routledge.

Trevarthen, C. (1980). The foundation of intersubjectivity: Development of interpersonal and cooperative understanding in infants. In D. Olsen (Ed.), *The social foundation of language and thought* (pp. 316–342). W. W. Norton & Co.

Trevarthen, C. (1998). The concept and foundations of infant intersubjectivity. In S. Bråten (Ed.), *Intersubjective communication and emotion in early ontogeny.* Cambridge University Press.

van der Kolk, B. (2015). *The body keeps the score: Brain, mind and body in the healing of trauma.* Penguin Books.

Winnicott, D. W. (1960). The theory of the parent-infant relationship. *International Journal of Psycho-analysis, 41,* 585–595.

Winnicott, D. W. (1972). Basis for self in body. *International Journal of Child Psychotherapy, 1*(1), 7–16.

Winnicott, D. W. (1982). *Playing and reality.* Tavistock Publications.

Woodhouse, S., Scott, J., Hepworth, A., & Cassidy, J. (2019). Secure base provision: A new approach to examining links between maternal caregiving and infant attachment. *Child Development,* 1–17. https://doi.org/10.1111/cdev.13224

Chapter 2

The Clinical Implications of Embodiment and Memory During Infancy

Maor, age 3, is at the hospital for neuroblastoma, where he is exhibiting severe stress behaviors leading into and during treatment days. These behaviors include disrupted sleep, food refusal, stranger anxiety, and resistant, phobic actions when attempting to enter the treatment room. Maor and his parents do not speak English, so even though we use some language during the session, many of our intentions are communicated nonverbally.

The dance and music therapists set up a large circle of chairs in a quiet area of the playroom to begin their weekly therapy group. This session features a table filled with music and DMT props, including lollipop drums, hand bells, rainbow-colored silk scarves, and a doll (wearing bandages from a previous child's play). As Maor and his parents enter, the music therapists sing a hello song, with one softly playing the guitar and the other keeping the beat with a drum, while I wave the rainbow scarf up and down in a welcoming gesture inside the circle. Dad sits across from Mom, who sits in a chair next to the music table. Maor places himself between Mom's legs, meekly leans over to pick up the lollipop drum and drumstick, and softly begins to beat the drum. Following his lead, I wave the scarf up and down, mirroring his beat. I glimpse Maor timidly glancing up at me. I respond with a gentle smile and nod. A slight smile crosses his face, momentarily acknowledging me, and he quickly looks back at Mom, who has also picked up a drum. Mom catches Maor's eye, playfully smiling, and glances at me, laughing kindly. Maor looks back at me with a bigger smile.

This exchange between us gives me the assurance that I need to try to expand our dialogue. I notice that Maor is slightly swaying side to side as he hits the drum. I mirror his sway, gently exaggerating it while moving my body and the scarf side to side, then swooping down and up. Maor, noticing this shift, takes the lead by crossing his foot behind his leg as he steps side to side with more strength. I exaggerate his strength, adding a firmer step, which Maor shifts into a marching step. Working in tandem with me, the music therapists seamlessly strengthen their beat, strumming the guitar and adding a more prominent tone to the musical mix. After picking up a hand bell and walking back and forth across the circle, Maor gives a bell to Dad, Mom, and me, one by one. There is a determined quality to his actions. I interpret this through my body, by standing taller as I march over to Maor, placing myself behind him. Dad and Mom follow suit, and Maor's steps become more staccato as he leads us around

DOI: 10.4324/9781003134800-3

the room. I now view Maor as an army general, getting his troops in order. I mark the sway of my arms with precision, and Maor, seeming to understand this analogy, looks back at us, his head a bit higher and a glimmer in his eye. He leads our procession around the room with a clear sense of purpose, looking back at us intermittently. I narrate our actions, stating he is the general and we are the soldiers in his command. The music therapists continue to attune to his every mood, becoming louder and softer, faster and slower, as our actions remain in step with his. Maor's smile broadens as his marching gets firmer and his understanding of the general and his army conceit is confirmed when he tests our allegiance by suddenly stopping his marching steps. We stop, too. Warmly, Maor looks at each of us as our bell ringing continues. The peaceful, beautiful, resonant musical interlude Maor has created through our wordless dancing interaction is palpable. As we pause, I am full of awe. Care and love fill the room. When Maor begins again, there is a new lightness in the quality of his actions as he transforms his downward stepping into a glide, shifting his weight up onto his right toe, counterbalancing by extending his other leg, floating it out to the left. This upward, lighter swinging movement is matched by his playful and more relaxed affect, which permeates the room.

Next comes the true essence of our dance: Maor brings us the silk rainbow scarf and we each take a corner of it, waving it up and down. With the lightness of our actions and the beauty of the billowing scarf, I am taken by an image of a rainbow after a storm. Maor completes this sense of calm and healing by including the baby doll. First, he removes her bandages, and then he cradles her in the scarf, assisting us in rocking her. As Mom joins, singing one of their favorite lullabies, I am filled with wonder and respect for the innocence and "old soulfulness" that exist simultaneously within this wise child. Through Maor's imaginative, innately artistic, spontaneous moving exploration, he is able to share his lived experience and transform its emotional power.

This session is a turning point in Maor's behavior. On this day, Maor enters his treatment, accompanied by me and his parents, with more emotional readiness. The nurse administering the treatment invites me to stay throughout the treatment to sustain the imagery developed in the session and to add soothing multisensory imagery to keep Maor focused on empowering and comforting sensations. Given his deep commitment to the general and soldiers metaphor, we build on this initial dance-play upon each return visit, providing Maor with both emotional expressivity and a level of control over his treatment experience that can continue to support him for the duration of his treatment. Upon completion of his treatment six months later, Mom sends us a note of gratitude, reflecting on how much our treatment helped the whole family navigate this difficult time in their lives, and highlighting the significant role his dance-play had in their ability to cope with his illness.

Clinical Discussion

This vignette illustrates how Maor is able to tell and transform his story through the lyrical and ineffable richness that comes from using the therapeutic arts of dance and music. It is both the quality of his embodied actions and the natural unfolding sequence of his dance-play story that enable us to gain visceral insight into his lived experience of medical treatment. His initial shy restraint shifts immediately into body–mind–emotional expression through his use of the drum and marching, grounding his felt experience. Maor's strong, downward rhythmic actions, supported by the adults who follow his cues, enable Maor to feel in control of some aspect of his life at a stressful time. Perception and action meet, creating a real and a metaphoric sense of strength. The intercorporeality of our experiences is evident as we all seamlessly attune to his actions. The moment-to-moment new image schemas that form through the specific qualitative elements of our dance – the strong, downward stamp of Maor's feet, coupled with the vertical emphasis of his body posture and the growing power of his march – provide the wordless acknowledgment that Maor needs. This enables him to transform his story of anguish into one of healing as we all follow his lead, using the flowing rainbow scarf to rock and sing to the baby doll, creating a fully embodied expression of Maor's inner experience.

This dance-play enables a transformation of the child's real-life experience, positively informing his developing concept of reality. This is also a good example of how the nonverbal embodied experience speaks for itself. Through the help of a translator, Maor's parents reflected on the significance of the metaphor of the general. They had realized that their child's difficult behaviors expressed his need for control, but it wasn't until they became his soldiers and experienced their son's transformation as the general that they truly felt how important it was for him to have some control within the context of his illness. This session was a turning point for them and Maor.

Introduction

As the fields of psychology, cognitive science, neuroscience, linguistics, philosophy, and affect neuroscience have abandoned Descartes's dualistic split between the mind and body, the term embodiment has become prominent in addressing the interrelatedness of body and mind. Although there is some variation in the theories and research focusing on the interpretations of the specific role of the body in human cognition, there is agreement with the general assumption that cognitive processes and self-knowledge are grounded in and inseparable from corporeal experience (Alessandroni, 2018). The term "embodiment" has grown beyond a simple neurological explanation of cognition to one that includes a broader inference about how the behaviors of the body, such as movement, postures, gestures, facial expressions and prosody, influence and simultaneously are influenced by the mind within physical and social contexts (Tschacher & Bergomi, 2011). The brain carries out functions with the body in an integrated way. This chapter provides a succinct synthesis of the various perspectives that are most relevant to our understanding of the impact of embodiment, felt experience, and memory in infancy as they impact the young pediatric patient's developing self.

The Role of the Body in Embodied Theories

Our bodies are always with us, and our felt experiences shape our perceptions and cognition. Embodied cognition states that the literal features of each individual's body and experience in their body – including body structures and positioning, composition and motor abilities – influence both perception and action, and thus shape one's personal cognitive experience (Gallagher, 2011). The actions we carry out through our body's explorations in the world orient and mold our conceptual systems (Lakoff & Johnson, 1999). Embodied simulation theory proposes that language understanding comes from our minds simulating the physical experience the words are describing. For example, our understanding of "up" in comparison to "down" comes from our sensation of verticality (Lakoff & Johnson, 2003). This occurs through the imaginative process of creating a virtual mental experience of perception and action without executing it.

Referencing the work of Gallese, Lakoff, and others in the field of cognitive semantics to explain the relationship between simulation and physical action, Alessandroni states: "Imagination and action have a neural substrate in common that links them directly and makes them functionally equivalent" (Alessandroni, 2018, p. 230). Indeed, the mirror neuron system (MNS) research of Gallese and colleagues (1996) has shown that sensorimotor information across several bodily modalities is triggered during specific reasoning, and linguistic understandings during the execution and observation of actions. Through the MNS, emotional states observed in one person are felt by the observer, enabling them to quickly and easily understand and feel the person's intentions and emotions. This automatic integration of another's behavior into our own (re)actions enables us to then predict the other's actions, supporting fast and flexible reactions during social exchanges (Jung & Sparenberg, 2012).

Imagination also involves perception and action. Concrete embodied experiences are the link in metaphoric analogies, and metaphor links embodied experience and conceptual understanding. Metaphors are created through recurring image schemas, constructed from bodily experiences that shape abstract conceptual thoughts. Our metaphoric thinking is a psychological function associated with and dependent on our corporeality (Alessandroni, 2018). Body-based image schemas include "front-back, in-out, near-far, pushing-pulling, supporting, balance" (Lakoff & Johnson, 1999, p. 36). Lakoff and Johnson provide the example that it is one's body-based, sensorimotor experience of verticality combined with subjective experience and judgment that link downwardness with the abstract concept of emotional sadness in the statement, "I am feeling down." While some theorists focus primarily on the individual's experience, others emphasize the interactive and social aspect of embodiment and its influence on social judgment (Gibbs, 2017). Embodied metaphoric associations have been found to have cross-cultural and cross-linguistic relevance. Examples include: "Intimacy is closeness – *We have a close relationship*; difficulties are burdens – *She's weighted down with responsibilities*; affection is warmth – *They greeted me warmly*; states are locations – *I'm close to being in a depression*" (Gibbs, 2017, p. 454, emphasis in original).

Merleau-Ponty's contributions, through the philosophical lens of phenomenology, have greatly influenced many contemporary perspectives on embodiment, including DMT. He states that the body provides knowledge and expression that is known only through its lived experience (Merleau-Ponty, 1945/2013). Merleau-Ponty views the body and the world as intertwined. His term "corporality" is explained from an experiential sense: We *are* a body, rather than the body simply being a physical object such that we *have* a body. Infants experience their bodies "both from within and as a 'thing.' This learning is of both 'what can *I* do' and 'what can *it* do.' Phenomenologists refer to these aspects of the 'lived body' . . . and the 'living body' . . . respectively" (de Haan et al., 2011, p. 138, emphasis in original). Merleau-Ponty uses the term "intercorporeality" to describe our pre-reflective bodily understanding of others during interactions that operate beyond our awareness. From birth, infants form subjective experiences when in relationship with another person, which creates recurring interactive patterns known as "schemes of being-with-another" (Stern, 1995, p. 80). These patterns include sensations, affects, actions, perceptions, motivations, thoughts, and social elements that are nonverbal and internally constructed from the experience of self when with another person who is separate from self. The infant begins to form representations within himself, about how he feels while in interaction with these specific others. Stern (2010, p. 11) and his colleagues (Boston-ChangeStudyGroup, 2010, p. 1) describe the embodied experiential nature of these interactions using the term "implicit relational knowing" to explain the way we know implicitly how to be with each other. Stern states that implicit knowledge is nonverbal, nonsymbolic, and nonconscious, and occurs through body-based experiences. The communication exists in the immediate moment through body-to-body dialogue, occurring without the need for words, and is unconscious, multisensory, and action based.

The Use of Embodiment and Embodied Concepts in Dance/Movement Therapy

Embodiment in DMT is grounded in psychological understanding of metaphor, consciousness, unconsciousness, nonconsciousness, and corporeality. In DMT, a fluid dynamic relationship exists between perception, action, emotion, movement, creativity and cognition, and "our existence is related to our own ways of experiencing" (Koch & Fischman, 2011, p. 66). The cornerstone of embodiment in DMT is the principle that one's sense of knowing comes from moving, which is fundamental, informing our sense of agency (Bloom, 2006; Sheets-Johnstone, 2011; Tortora, 2013). Koch (2011), a dance therapist and researcher in the field, highlights the expressive, creative, and artistic facets of DMT in her definition of embodiment as integral and in unique aspects of DMT methodology. The artistic and aesthetic aspects of personal creative dance and movement expression create a somatic narrative that is integral to the transformative process of healing (Eberhard-Kaechele, 2012). A somatic narrative comes from a "bottom-up" body and sensorimotor information-processing approach, denoting that physical- and movement-based impulses, including interoceptive sensations, precede and inform thought, and are the basis for higher cognitive processing (Erickson, 2021).

Building upon this definition of embodiment, dance therapists also use the term embodied to describe when a person is in a state of full engagement with body, mind, and emotion. This creates a rich felt experience for the mover and observer, communicating a sense of commitment to the moment as the mover's feelings are conveyed through their body actions. This is especially evident, for example, when watching a dance performance: When the dancer's actions are imbued with deep emotion, it seems as if every cell in the performer's body is engaged in communicating. The audience is captivated on visceral, somatic, and emotional levels. Conversely, when a mover is disembodied, a feeling of disengagement is conveyed. A sense of connection to self is missing. The mover appears to be cut off from his emotions, severing the body from the mind and feelings, lacking presence. In its extreme, this type of detachment is similar to dissociation in psychoanalysis. Being disembodied is also a state of being, because, at times, as implied by Winnicott (1987, p. 91), moving from a place of full body–mind–emotional connectedness may be too powerful or triggering, and one becomes "unavailable to consciousness."

Embodiment, the Present Moment, and Implicit and Explicit Memory

Merleau-Ponty's concept of the present moment is pertinent to our discussion of embodiment. He views the present moment as a place where we arrive freshly and suddenly. It may include a memory, a novel thought, or a new perception that, in the immediacy of the moment, is intuitive and not necessarily in our consciousness. Influenced by this perspective, the fields of psychology and psychoanalysis have explored the experience of the present moment as a subjective experience in everyday life and the therapeutic relationship. Stern (2004, p. 26) discusses how the present moment has a temporal phrasing quality that is a "flowing whole occurring during a now" moment, that includes the past and the unfolding future. He states that the past may echo in the present moment, overshadowing the present if its shadow is too strong. The future can equally hold the present moment hostage, but

> the present moment is never totally eclipsed by the past nor fully erased by the future. It retains a form of its own while being influenced by what went before and what comes after. Also, it determines the shape of the past that is brought forward into the present and the outlines of the imagined future. This trialogue between past, present, and future occurs almost continuously from moment to moment in art, life, and psychotherapy.
>
> (Stern, 2004, p. 31)

The immediacy of the present moment as a concretization of the past, present, and future also brings us to Winnicott. Winnicott's (1987, p. 91) reference to the continuity of life – that "nothing that has been part of an individual's life experience is lost or can ever be lost" – supports the DMT perspective that our bodies are a map of our experiences, including preverbal experience. The integrating of the body and the mind creates a body–mind–emotional continuum that begins at or even prior to birth and informs the infant's core self from a reality-based perception (Tortora, 2019). It leads to the understanding that our bodies hold our experiences and are expressed through our actions. As suggested by Winnicott, and more recently demonstrated in trauma research, some experiences are felt and stay in our awareness; but there are also experiences, especially preverbal, difficult, or traumatic ones, that are held out of awareness and stored deeply in the body (van der Kolk, 2015). The terms implicit or procedural memory are used in cognitive psychology to describe memories that are nonconscious, which "sink into implicit unconscious knowing" and are, in essence, inscribed into body memory through our moving, sensing, sensorimotor, and felt experience (Fuchs, 2012, p. 13). Implicit memories are nonverbal, in contrast to declarative or explicit memories that remain conscious. The cognitive sciences once viewed implicit and explicit memory as polarized, but more recent work, especially in trauma recovery, suggests a more complex, fluid relationship between them (Fuchs, 2012; Gaensbauer, 2011). Explicit memories may arise through body re-enactments of implicit body memories.

Creating Verbal and Embodied Coherent Narratives

Susan Coates, a psychoanalyst who treats young children and trauma, provides three clinical case studies that examine how quite early traumatic events experienced by preverbal children are storied in memory. Specifically, her interest is in whether a child has the capacity for symbolic representation and interpretation of these events later in treatment, and the role of the attachment relationship in the resolution of the trauma (Coates, 2016). Her studies demonstrate that neonates, infants, and toddlers do have the capacity to experience intense pain, to interpret events as harrowing and life threatening, and to demonstrate traumatic symptoms. These events can be symbolically held in the child's memory, affecting later behaviors and learning. Children are capable of creating age-related symbolic representations of the trauma, and the successful or unsuccessful resolution of the trauma can be deeply connected to the quality and function of the attachment system.

In his clinical work, psychiatrist Ted Gaensbauer confirms Winnicott's statement: that "nothing that has been part of an individual's life experience is lost or can ever be lost" (Winnicott, 1987, pp. 90–91) by showing how preverbal trauma, either experienced or witnessed, is represented in the behavior and traumatic re-enactment play schemes of infants, toddlers, and children. Gaensbauer's detailed close observation and documentation of young children's nonverbal and verbal behaviors reveal how sensory experiences and motor actions are linked and become imprinted (Gaensbauer, 2002, 2014). He developed the term "perceptual-cognitive-affective-sensory-motor schemata" to explain how experiences are organized and represented through actions (Gaensbauer, 2004, p. 29). This concept describes how preverbal and sensory-based memory form on multiple levels through emotional and somatic experiences that can later manifest through clinical symptoms and atypical behaviors in childhood, including hyper- and hypo-arousal states, anxiety, phobias, nightmares and night terrors, avoidance of stimuli related to the traumatic event, and distress at reminders acting as triggers of the experience. As stated by Gaensbauer (2004, p. 29), "The intimate coupling between sensory experiences and motoric actions that replicate these experiences provides important depth to our understanding of the representations that underlie reenactment behavior," because "the child's verbal and nonverbal understanding is separate from their conscious and unconscious expressions of their traumas" Gaensbauer (2018).

Gaensbauer also references the role of the MNS in creating enduring internal representations that become memories that are "burned in" on multiple motor, sensory, and affective modalities, which can be activated long after the original event(s) occurred (Gaensbauer, 2011). Significant for the theme of this book, Gaensbauer identifies the infant's capacity from birth for imitation (Meltzoff & Moore, 1997) as an example of the MNS operating from the start, stating that the younger the child, the more susceptible they are to undiluted imitative behavior, such as traumatic modeling, without the capacity for higher-level associative and integrative processing.

Young children can experience enduring representations of a trauma which can last for weeks, months, and even years, as manifested through recognition of traumatic reminders, emotional and behavioral reliving including traumatic re-enactment, avoidance of stimuli associated with the trauma, dominance of traumatic themes, and many other symptoms.

(Gaensbauer, 2014)

The MNS provides a means of explaining the deep emotional, somatic, and visceral ways in which dance therapists gain insight into the baby's and parent's experience when moving and witnessing them during non-verbal dance and movement-oriented therapeutic explorations. Attending to their perceptive and interoceptive experiences, dance therapists match and complement the baby's and parents' affective expressions and actions to come to know their somatic and psychological state. Through movement exchanges, they learn with the mover how their body and signature movement styles reveal, hold, and express their past and current experiences.

It is through the process of facilitating this level of embodied connection that dance therapists support their patients to use their bodies to tell their stories. Working from the understanding that the body naturally creates a nonverbal and somatic narrative through movement in its own nonlinear way, we use techniques that heighten the expression of this embedding narrative through activities that include body awareness and connectedness, sensorial/interoceptive sensing, and enactment through movement and dance (Caldwell, 2014; Gallagher & Hutto, 2019). Similar to the coherent verbal narratives created in the therapeutic re-enactment play techniques of Gaensbauer and Coates, dance therapists strive to support their patients to create "embodied coherent narratives" (Tortora, 2019, p. 6). Initially, these embodied narratives can occur as movement and sensation fragments, sequences, and enactments without obvious associations and meanings. In their own time, as they are given room to be expressed, supported, and engaged in dialogue within the therapeutic movement environment, they become organized and incorporated, establishing their own body coherence and communicability. Through this process the observant dance therapist detects their communicative potential, viewing them as movement metaphors that may remain on the somatic level for resolution or facilitate a verbal narrative. In the session, interactive dance and movement activities function on concrete and metaphoric levels, facilitating the development of image schemas that stimulate the body and mind. By honoring the felt experience, fueled by interoceptive sensations that align actions with feelings, embodied coherent narratives integrate verbal storytelling and non-verbal and somatic experiences that occur on a primary processing level. As stated by Caldwell (2016, p. 230), "Being able to tell one's story after or at the same time as one moves, it can result in profound integration on brain, body, and relational levels."

Specifically when working with children therapeutically, Tortora (2006, p. 289) uses the term "dance-play" to describe the integration of activities that incorporate the body, movement, dance, and play. "Dance" emphasizes the fluid nonverbal expressivity of the body and somatic experience, while "play" emphasizes the use of play elements that naturally enter the interaction when working with children. What differentiates dance-play interventions from recreational play and play-therapy methods is the focus on the body and the experience of the body as the central therapeutic tool. With the addition of a dance lens, we can consider how dance elements – such as rhythm, phrasing, spatial placement, and weight shifting – can transform the actions that create deeper embodied symbolic meaning, which may or may not need verbal interpretation for healing.

Clinical Implications for the Young Baby's Lived Experience

The baby's experience of his physical body during a medical illness, which restricts his natural inclinations for active exploration, creates a very specific personal lived experience. Furthermore, despite extreme care, medical treatment unavoidably includes painful procedures, which the young child often perceives as more frightening than the disease itself. The medical team must treat the young body, being the physical object that it is, to perform procedures required to cure a potentially life-threatening illness. Hence, we must always consider the lived experience of the baby in his body, the body as a lived-in body *and* a living body, while being sensitive to residual emotional "scars," conscious or unconscious, as a result of the object experience. This means we must include psychological care in the treatment plan. The body is the baby's first locus of experience and expression from which meaning is generated through interactions with the world, and most importantly, the significant people in the baby's world. As in Chapter 1's discussion of Tortora's sense of body concept, it is the baby's experience of her body in dynamic interaction with the world around her that provides awareness of who she is and how she organizes her experiences. The study of embodiment includes the intersubjective interactions between infants and their primary caregivers that occur from birth. Infants are born with mental structures to engage and emotionally connect with the feeling states of others. Intersubjective interactions involving facial expressions, gestures, postures, and full-body actions are considered the neural foundations of enactive social perception and motor intentions, which go beyond simple simulation or mimicking of actions and mental states (Gallagher, 2011).

Embodiment happens through social experiences. Sebanz and colleagues Jung and Sparenberg (2012, p. 148) state that it is through joint actions defined as "any form of social interaction whereby two or more individuals coordinate their actions in space and time to bring about a change in the environment" that one gets to know oneself and other. The communicative nature of social interactions causes us to modify our cognitive perceptions to successfully engage with others. The embodiment research speaks of the natural pull to rhythmically coordinate during social interactions, which provides the foundation for Malloch and Trevarthen's communicative musicality concept, discussed in Chapter 1. Individuals do not gain a conceptualization of self and an understanding of an emotional self in a vacuum; rather, it is through coordinated interactive exchanges that an individual internalizes perspectives of others and develops an embodied conceptualization of self as distinct from other.

Conclusions

This chapter focuses on embodiment and infancy memory, keeping the baby's bodily sensed and lived experience in mind so we can think about how this awareness can inform how we treat the young pediatric patient within the context of their family. Babies' social and emotional development, as they are felt, held, and expressed through their embodied experiences, must be considered side by side, especially during an infant's journey with medical illness. Healing requires us to "speak the unspeakable" (Lieberman, 2021), but to fully heal, we must also embody the wordless experiences that are felt and held in the body. This includes honoring and preserving the caregiver-infant attachment relationship so it can be soothing and organizing for the infant. In this chapter we synthesize theoretical and empirical findings, building bridges between neuroscience, philosophy, linguistics, traditional cognitive and developmental psychology and somatic psychology, linking felt experience, cognition, and psychological understanding, to make associations between how babies' physical experiences of their bodies during medical treatment inform their budding corporeal sensibility, emotional and social relationships, and abstract concepts of reality. This chapter asks: What unique, dynamic recurring patterns might form during the young child's real-life medical experiences that occur over extended periods of time? How might these interactive patterns deeply influence the child's body-based image schemas, informing the mapping of more traditional interpretative metaphors? For example, what happens when closeness and warmth are associated with pain and being restrained rather than comfort and caring?

The aesthetic and expressive elements of DMT activities support the patient to create new dynamic patterns, linking motor actions, perceptions, affect, and memories with the potential to shape new cognitive understandings and memories. The intrinsic body, movement, and nonverbal aspects of DMT, coupled with the very young child's natural propensity for creative expressive dance and movement, uniquely position

DMT as an effective treatment method that can support a child to synthesize potentially traumatic aspects of their medical experience *while* they are undergoing medical treatment. It is our hope that providing these young children with the ability to express their feelings in treatment, within the context of an embodied psychotherapeutic milieu, can create perceptual-cognitive-affective-sensory-motor schemata that foster expressivity and empowerment, instead of internalized representations of trauma (Tortora, 2019).

Again, Winnicott's (1987, pp. 90–91) words come to mind to explain this concept:

> The basis of all theories about human development is continuity, the line of life, which presumably starts before the baby's actual birth; continuity which carries with it the idea that nothing that has been part of an individual's experience is lost or can ever be lost to that individual, even if in various complex ways it should and does become unavailable to consciousness . . . . It will be observed that I am taking you to a place where verbalization has no meaning.

Through this healing dance of connection to self and others, perhaps we can find expression for those experiences that are lost to consciousness, creating a fully embodied "continuity" through "the line of life" that needs no words to be experienced, as Winnicott illuminates.

References

Alessandroni, N. (2018). Varieties of embodiment in cognitive science. *Theory & Psychology*, *28*(2), 227–248. https://doi.org/10.1177/0959354317745589

Bloom, K. (2006). *The embodied self: Movement and psychoanalysis.* Karnac.

BostonChangeStudyGroup. (2010). *Change in psychotherapy: A unifying paradigm.* W. W. Norton.

Caldwell, C. (2014). Mindfulness and bodyfulness: A new paradigm. *Journal of Contemplative Inquiry*, 77–96.

Caldwell, C. (2016). Body identity development: Definitions and discussions. *Body, Movement and Dance in Psychotherapy*, *11*(4), 220–234. https://doi.org/10.1080/17432979.1145141

Coates, S. (2016). Can babies remember trauma? Symbolic forms of representation in traumatized infants. *The Journal of the American Psychoanalytic Association*, *64*(4), 751–776. https://doi.org/doi.org/10.1177/0003065116659443

de Haan, S., De Jaegher, H., Fuchs, T., & Mayers, A. (2011). Expanding perspectives: The interactive development of perspective-taking in early childhood. In W. Tschacher & C. Bergomi (Eds.), *The Implications of embodiment: Cognition and communication* (pp. 129–147). Imprint Academic.

Eberhard-Kaechele, M. (2012). Memory, metaphor, mirroring and trauma. In S. Koch, T. Fuchs, M. Summa, & C. Muller (Eds.), *Body memory, metaphor and movement* (pp. 267–287). John Bejamins Publishing Company.

Erickson, L. (2021). Sensing the body: A dance/movement therapy model of embodied identity development. *Body, Movement and Dance in Psychotherapy, 16*(3), 202–217. https://doi.org/10.1080/17432979.2020.1850524

Fuchs, T. (2012). The phenomenology of body memory. In S. Koch, T. Fuchs, M. Summa, & C. Muller (Eds.), *Body memory, metaphor and movement* (pp. 9–22). John Bejamins Publishing Company.

Gaensbauer, T. (2002). Representations of trauma in infancy: Clinical and theoretical implications for the understanding of early memory. *Infant Mental Health Journal, 23*(3), 259–277.

Gaensbauer, T. (2004). Telling their stories: Representation and reenactment of traumatic experiences occurring in the first year of life. *Zero to Three, 24*(5), 25–31.

Gaensbauer, T. (2011). Embodied simulation, mirror neurons, and the reenactment of trauma in early childhood. *Neuropsychoanalysis, 13*(1), 91–108.

Gaensbauer, T. (2014, January 8). *Telling their stories: Representation and reenactment of early traumatic experiences.* Ways of Seeing International Webinar.

Gaensbauer, T. (2018, November 7). Personal communication [Interview].

Gallagher, S. (2011). Interpretations of embodied cognition. In W. Tschacher & C. Bergomi (Eds.), *The implications of embodiment: Cognition and communication* (pp. 59–68). Imprint Academic.

Gallagher, S., & Hutto, D. (2019). Narratives in embodied therapeutic practice: Getting the story straight. In H. Payne, S. Koch, J. Tantia, & T. Fuchs (Eds.), *The Routledge international handbook of embodied perspectives in psychotherapy* (pp. 28–39). Routledge.

Gallese, V., Fadiga, L., Fogassi, L., & Rizzolatti, G. (1996). Action recognition in the premotor cortex. *Brain, 119*(Pt 2), 593–609.

Gibbs, R. (2017). Embodiment. In B. Dancygier (Ed.), *The Cambridge handbook of cognitive linguistics* (pp. 449–462). Cambridge University Press. https://doi.org/10.1017/9781316339732

Jung, C., & Sparenberg, P. (2012). Cognitive perspectives on embodiment. In S. Koch, T. Fuchs, M. Summa, & C. Muller (Eds.), *Body memory, metaphor and movement* (pp. 141–154). John Bejamins Publishing Company.

Koch, S. (2011). Basic body rhythms: From individual to interpersonal movement feedback. In W. Tschacher & C. Bergomi (Eds.), *The implications of embodiment: Cognition and communication* (pp. 151–171). Imprint Academic.

Koch, S., & Fischman, D. (2011). Embodied enactive dance/movement therapy. *American Journal of Dance Therapy, 33*, 57–32.

Lakoff, G., & Johnson, M. (1999). *Philosophy in the flesh: The embodied mind and its challenge to western thought.* Basic Books.

Lakoff, G., & Johnson, M. (2003). *Metaphors we live.* University of Chicago Press.

Lieberman, A. (2021, March 8). *Promoting child-parent symbolic play to repair early trauma* The Spectrum of Play, Online Conference. https://profectum.org/2021-conference-spectrum-play/

Meltzoff, A., & Moore, M. (1997). Explaining facial imitation: A theoretical model. *Early Development Parent, 6*, 179–192. https://doi.org/10.1002/(SICI)1099-0917(199709/12)6:3/4<179::AID-EDP157>3.0.CO;2-R

Merleau-Ponty, M. (1945/2013). *Phenomenology of perception.* Routledge.

Sheets-Johnstone, M. (2011). *The primacy of movement* (2nd ed.). John Benjamin's Publishing Company.

Stern, D. (1995). *The motherhood constellation: A unified view of parent-infant psychotherapy.* Basic Books Inc.

Stern, D. (2004). *The present moment in psychotherapy and everyday life*. W. W. Norton & Company.

Stern, D. (2010). *Forms of vitality: Exploring dynamic experiences in psychology, the arts, psychotherapy, and development*. Oxford University Press.

Tortora, S. (2006). *The dancing dialogue: Using the communicative power of movement with young children*. Paul H. Brookes Publishing Company.

Tortora, S. (2013). The essential role of the body in the parent-infant relationship: Nonverbal analysis of attachment. In J. F. Bettmann (Ed.), *Attachment-based clinical social work with children and adolescents* (pp. 141–164). Springer.

Tortora, S. (2019). Children are born to dance! Pediatric medical dance/movement therapy: The view from integrative pediatric oncology. *Children, 6*(14), 1–27. https://doi.org/10.3390/children6010014

Tschacher, W., & Bergomi, C. (2011). Introduction. In W. Tschacher & C. Bergomi (Eds.), *The Implications of embodiment: Cognition and communication* (pp. vii–x). Imprint Academic.

van der Kolk, B. (2015). *The body keeps the score: Brain, mind and body in the healing of trauma*. Penguin Books.

Winnicott, D. W. (1987). *Babies and their mothers*. Addison-Wesley Publishing Company, Inc.

Chapter 3

Principles of Pediatric Medical Dance/Movement Therapy

Introduction

When introducing DMT to a caregiver or medical professional, the dance therapist is often asked, "How can a baby dance if they cannot move and are feeling so sick?" Throughout this book, we provide vignettes illustrating the use of DMT with very young children. In this chapter, we define the specific principles and mechanisms of DMT – including its emergence as a psychotherapeutic field and specific influences from related fields – to explain its application as a pediatric medical treatment modality and an integral feature of integrative medicine's support services (Tortora, 2015a, 2016, 2019).

Defining "Dance" in Dance/Movement Therapy – Historic and Current

Before we can explain how the practice of DMT has grown to include working with the youngest patients, it is important to understand its historic origins as it grew from the self-expressive explorations of dancers into a psychotherapeutic modality and how the profession defines the field. According to the American Dance Therapy Association (ADTA), DMT is "the psychotherapeutic use of movement to promote emotional, social, cognitive, and physical integration of the individual, for the purpose of improving health and well-being" (ADTA, 2021). The term "dance" in the name evokes many references that include literal and metaphoric uses of dance. In contemporary DMT, dance has come to be one of many nonverbal, movement- and body-based activities employed in the effort to understand the patient's psychological experience. Dance has a breadth and depth of meaning that includes the observation and use of everyday actions, play, movement, dance, body awareness, breath awareness, guided imagery, and mindfulness activities. A prominent feature of DMT is understanding the body and body actions as key nonverbal sources of information about feeling states, which may be conscious or unconscious. Gray, a dance therapist

DOI: 10.4324/9781003134800-4

who specializes in trauma work, aptly describes the prominent role dance plays in development and healing:

> If movement is a primary language, then dance is the creative expression of our first language . . . . [The] sequential developmental movement process becomes the neurosequential, sensorimotor, somatically based foundation of our sensing, feeling, thinking, and action . . . . If we describe the developmental trajectory of childhood as an embodied, creative process, then the disruption of this process instigated by wounding, trauma, or disease can only be restored somatically and creatively.
>
> (Gray & Porges, 2017, pp. 103–104)

Unique to DMT is the artistic use and understanding of motion to express and communicate emotion within the safety of a psychotherapeutic milieu. The early DMT innovators looked toward the historic role of dance in all ancient and contemporary cultures as a form of medicine, cultural identity, and personal expression, and then built upon these uses as they worked through the lens of emerging psychological fields (Bernstein, 1979). These early dance therapists worked with adult hospitalized patients with mental health conditions, including anxiety, depression, and "the normal, functioning neurotic" (Levy, 2005, p. 34). The original dance therapists working with children and youth saw them in hospitalized, institutional, and special education settings, primarily addressing conditions such as autism spectrum disorder (ASD), visual impairment, trauma from sexual abuse, attachment disorders, and physical and learning difficulties (Levy, 1995, 2005). The field of dance/movement therapy emerged from early collaborative experiences with psychiatry and special education, creating a distinction between dance as a recreational activity and a psychotherapeutic modality.

Distinction Between Dance/Movement Therapy and Other Movement, Somatic, and Mindfulness Fields

This distinction is important to understand because the sometimes playful, physical nature of a DMT session can belie the depth of the emotional content being explored. The phrase "psychotherapeutic use of movement" in the ADTA definition is crucial, for DMT is often confused with other movement- and mind/body-focused activities used to promote wellness, including yoga, relaxation, guided imagery, mindfulness, contemporary dance, improvisation, therapeutic dance, and martial arts. These programs focus on physical-skill training taught by a professional teacher in the specific field, and often involve learning dance choreography, yoga postures, martial arts moves, or meditative and breathing techniques to focus one's attention. These excellent skills support the patient in feeling a sense of competence and control in their body. Many dance/movement therapists have training in and include skills from these techniques as part of their therapeutic repertoire, especially when working in medical DMT (Goodill, 2005).

What differentiates DMT is that it is a form of psychotherapy with an added experiential, physical, creative arts focus. Dance/movement therapists view the body, body actions, sensations, and behaviors as a rich source of nonverbal psychic material. The therapist creates body, dance, and movement activities to support embodied discoveries along the body–mind–emotional continuum, within the context of the psychotherapeutic container created by the therapist witnessing and moving with the patient (Pallaro, 1999; Tortora, 2015b). These aesthetic and deeply personal creative explorations also distinguish DMT from other mindfulness and body-oriented psychotherapeutic approaches. The physical activities a patient engages in are designed to convey emotions. All dance- and movement-based activities are set within the context of the artistic expression of the body. During these activities, the therapist discerns the psychological connections between nonverbal and verbal expressions to support further expression. Through these embodied emotive explorations, the patient develops coping skills. This embodied approach supports patients to express their nonverbal felt experiences through sensorial emotionally rich activities developed around personal themes. Conducted as individual or group sessions, these innovative explorations foster conscious and unconscious self-understandings that can transform into verbalizations, cognitive understandings, and behavioral changes in daily life (Koch & Fischman, 2011). Since the body and actions are the primary source of expression, interaction, and learning, the central nonverbal and bodily aspect of the treatment is a natural fit for preverbal and early childhood.

Embodied Countertransference to the Parents and Young Child with Medical Illness

The extensive, physically active role the dance/movement therapist plays in this treatment places the dance therapist's own body at the heart of the treatment method (Hervey, 2007; Pallaro, 1999). Similar to the way verbal therapists attend to their words as countertransferential material, dance/movement therapists keenly attend to their own actions, regarding their bodies as tools in the therapeutic process to understand their embodied countertransference (Bloom, 2006; Koch & Fischman, 2011). Embodied countertransference refers to the dance therapist's lived body experience. Attuning to personal responses on a body, mind, and emotional level within the context of the therapeutic relationship influences how the dance therapist understands the patient's experience and paces the session. This becomes especially important in light of medical procedures a young child experiences that may trigger physically painful, unconscious associations in the therapist and the parents, too.

The specific body, mind, and emotional components of embodied countertransference the dance therapist pays attention to and analyzes are described in detail in another publication (Tortora, 2006) and are outlined here. "Witnessing" relates to tracking the immediate associations, images, thoughts, and personal and theoretical references that come to mind. "Kinesthetic seeing" is used to describe how the therapist tracks her somatic, kinesthetic, sensorial, and interoceptive body responses. "Kinesthetic empathy" involves tracking emotional responses, including personal triggers that may influence how the therapist interprets and responds to the patient and family members.

These aspects of embodied countertransference shed light on the therapist's conscious and unconscious bias developed through her own ethnic, cultural, and personal experiences. The therapist's own lens will influence their felt experience; this in turn affects how they perceive, respond to, and support the therapeutic milieu, and the specific dance and movement-based activities that unfold in the session. Embodied ethical decision-making (EEDM), developed by Harvey, a dance therapist working in mental health care, provides specific steps for the therapist to uncover cultural and ethical bias that may arise in their bodily responses (Hervey, 2007; Roberts, 2021). Roberts (2021), also a dance therapist working in mental health care, recently adapted this framework, developing a method based on active multicultural diversity (AMD) that furthers ethical decision-making via a process that enables the therapist to become aware of and act upon the role culture plays in their movement-based suggestions within the context of the patient's situation. The details of both valuable methods go beyond the focus of this book, but one salient aspect pertaining to embodied countertransference in the pediatric setting includes attending to how the nonverbal expression styles of each member of the dancing/movement dialogue reveal pertinent information about their sociocultural experience, understanding, and belief system related to medical illness. The goal is to use this information, revealed in part through nonverbal expression, to create a sense of respect, collaboration, mutuality, and empowerment as the patient and caregivers feel seen through the movement exchange. The dance therapist accomplishes this by considering how the sociocultural contexts of the children and families, and the lens of DMT, influence their responses, family dynamics, understandings, and reactions to medical illness as they unfold throughout treatment.

The Application of DMT to Medical and Pediatric Settings

Dr. Sherry Goodill (2005), a former president of the ADTA, was the first dance therapist in the United States to gather in one publication all the work being done in the then-emerging field of medical dance/movement therapy. She helped define medical DMT, incorporating treatment goals to address concerns particular to medical illness, such as improving body awareness and body-self image, increasing self-care, improving quality of life, increasing vitality and energy, building a sense of resilience and hope, reducing depression and anxiety, stress management, the development of pain management techniques, decreasing fatigue, improving social support and the ability to receive social support, and learning to accept the unpredictability of life (Goodill, 2018; Koch et al., 2014; Madden et al., 2010; Tortora, 2019).

Pediatric medical DMT is a little known yet growing application of the field (Cohen & Walco, 1999; Goodill, 2005; Tortora, 2019; Zilius, 2010). This treatment serves pediatric patients suffering from acute, life-threatening, or chronic medically based conditions in inpatient and outpatient hospital settings, pediatric intensive care units (PICUs), private practice clinics, and hospice (Cohen, 1996; Goodill & Morningstar, 1993). Among the medical conditions addressed are prematurity and other pre- and perinatal birth-related conditions, chronic pain, scoliosis, cancer, migraines, asthma, heart disease, Tourette's syndrome and other neurological disorders, physical accidents, and heart disease. In hospital settings, this application most often occurs within the context of child-life or integrative medicine (Cohen, 2000; Tortora, 2019). For an overview of pediatric medical DMT's current prevalence and application worldwide, which goes beyond the scope of this book, see Tortora (2019).

Goodill and Morningstar (1993) published one of the earliest articles about pediatric medical DMT. It emphasizes how the combined use of movement as the primary communication, coupled with the creative process, enables the child with medical illness to explore their body image through symbolic expression. Medical treatment can greatly change one's body functioning, which in turn will affect the pediatric patient's body image. Childhood is a time when body image is already dynamic. Dance and actively using our bodies to explore the world are innate pleasures of this time of life. Movement is the primary way a child learns about her surroundings. Creative dance expression and active movement discoveries provide a sense of body control and expression for the young child. The ability to playfully participate in childhood activities is often compromised during serious medical illness. This can seriously impede a sense of mastery, replacing it with a feeling for the child that her body and disease are out of her control. This feeling has been compared to a loss of agency and disempowerment for patients, and it can trigger subsequent stress physiology that occurs when facing a threatening or traumatic life event (Cloitre et al., 2009; Nir, 1985; Schechter, 2017; Terr, 1992). During this early stage of development, DMT provides a physical avenue of exploration and expression of the young patient's body experience. This enables the pediatric patient to stay in touch with a central layer of emerging selfhood within the context of her medical illness (Mendelsohn, 1999).

As discussed in Chapter 2, the expressive features of DMT offer the pediatric patient an opportunity to eradicate a sense of helplessness by building a nonverbal narrative during the course of treatment, as an "embodied coherent narrative," that can prevent or heal the traumatic effects of the medical experience (Tortora, 2019, p. 22). An embodied coherent narrative, which is rich in empowering multisensory and interoceptive sensations, integrates verbal and nonverbal means of expression that can have a restorative and healing effect. Creating a sense of mastery and control over difficult life events is a core element of many trauma treatments (Cloitre et al., 2009; Levine & Kline, 2008; Levine, 2012; Minde, 2000; van der Kolk, 2015). In addition to repairing a sense of helplessness, DMT can change the fraught body image to one of health, comfort, and strength (Cohen, 1999). This focus supports adjusting to and acceptance of the child's body rather than focusing on possible dysfunctions caused by disease.

As stated by Madden and her colleagues in their research about DMT and other creative arts therapies with children with brain tumors undergoing chemotherapy,

> By using creative expression, a child or adolescent with cancer can express feelings about the course of the disease and tumultuous treatment through dance/movement, music, and art. This outlet allows the patient to creatively and kinesthetically process the assaults of cancer and its treatment, and thus establish a stronger sense of self and improved quality of life.
>
> (Madden et al., 2010, p. 133)

Susan Rizzo Vincent, the founder of the Andréa Rizzo Foundation, an organization that funds many pediatric oncology DMT programs in the United States, including the program Tortora created, best summarizes the focus of pediatric medical DMT:

> I have a nice, simple way of describing what dance/movement therapy is [via the acronym ART]: A [for how] the dance/movement therapist ACCESSES emotions like fear, anxiety, anger that a child with cancer may be feeling through dance and movement expression, usually with the child taking the lead; R [for how] the emotions are RELEASED through this movement (we all know how good it [can] feel to dance out our frustrations); T [for how] TRANSFORMATION takes place, physically and emotionally, through dance and movement, giving the child new ways to express themselves and to cope.
>
> (Tortora, 2019, p. 6)

The following vignette, featuring Tommy, a 3.5-year-old boy with leukemia, exemplifies ART.

> As usual, I warmly greet Tommy to begin our DMT session; however, Tommy is not his usual smiley self, eager to dance. He is withdrawn and avoids my gaze. He is cuddled in bed on Dad's lap, holding his tense body in a tight ball, molding into Dad's embrace. With compassion, I tell Tommy, "Oh, I see, you are so cozy with Daddy and are not ready to dance yet. I'll give you some time before we begin." As I direct my attention to Dad, I notice Tommy slightly soften his tight posture. Dad tells me that Tommy has been like this all week, and he cannot get Tommy to engage in anything. Dad also says that his blood platelet count has dropped again, so they will not be going home as expected. As Dad shares this news, Tommy abruptly tenses his whole body, pressing his weight into Dad. I wonder to myself if this non-verbal action reveals an underlying emotion, silently taking out my soft feeling balls with printed images of mad, sad, happy, scared, and worried expressions. From the corner of my eye, I notice Tommy looks at the balls, so I gently roll them toward him on his bed. They settle in a group at his feet. I pause, holding my body quietly, softly gazing at Tommy. He slowly extends his right leg, kicking the red "angry" ball off the bed, as if tossing it away. Brushing the other balls to the side, I pick up the red ball and, matching the quality of his kick, roll it back to him. As we continue, his pause and kick turn into a focused exchange, and our passing the ball becomes a rhythmic game with direction and strength. I match the rhythm, putting on his favorite song. Tommy immediately sits up, independent of Dad, and bounces to the beat. I gently throw the ball to him; he catches it and throws it back. Next, I throw the ball to Dad, and soon a three-way catching game in rhythm to the music develops. As Tommy gets his feelings out through this wordless, spontaneous dance-game, we all experience his mood shift from tense and angry to playful. Dad smiles with gratitude. After the game, Dad and I discuss how he feels about needing to stay in the hospital longer, how sensitive Tommy is to his reactions, and how important it is to have Dad engage with us in our dance-play.

Clinical Discussion

When reading about Tommy's case, we may wonder whether he is depressed or simply reacting to his father's sadness. It is important to make this distinction, because the answer will implicate a different intervention. And that answer is evident when we see how easily Tommy engages and his mood brightens during the dance-play. If he was depressed, he would not have reacted so positively and so quickly. He is angry, but feels better when the therapist gives him the opportunity to enact his anger. Tortora's task is multifaceted: First, she must "sense the essence in the air," defined as the emotional mood and tension level in the room that can be felt and experienced, but initially it may not be spoken about (Tortora, 2006, p. 241); next, she must determine how to create an activity that holds the parent's emotional vulnerability and difficulty while enabling Tommy to express his angry and frustrated feelings. This is a very common dynamic between children and their parents at the hospital. Despite Dad's attempt to present a positive disposition to Tommy, he is understandably very disappointed that they are not going home. As Tommy enacts his emotions through the dance-play, Tortora verbalizes, "Wow, look how strong your feelings are! It is so good to get your angry feelings out!" Enabling the therapist to be the recipient of Tommy's difficult mood, with Dad as the observer, creates a safe place for Tommy's difficult feelings to be expressed, making the unspeakable speakable, without the feelings being directed at Dad. This also gives Dad a much-needed moment to reflect on his own feelings. After Tommy has the chance to express his true feelings, his mood lightens. Including Dad in the play at this point shifts their interaction from sullen to playful, and actively supports the expression of feelings for them both. Over time, as Dad becomes more comfortable holding Tommy's difficult emotions, he can better navigate Tommy's behaviors reflecting his distress.

Specific Intervention Strategies in DMT with Very Young Children with Medical Illness

These strategies, summarized in Figure 3.1, begin with the dance therapist, who operates from the perspective that all nonverbal behaviors have the potential to be a form of meaningful communication, providing a window into how the child and caregivers are responding to their experiences. To view all actions as potential communication, one must pay close attention to the unique nonverbal cues of the child and caregivers, as well as the therapist's own embodied countertransference experience. Dance therapy nonverbal analysis training includes skills in observing what the mover is doing and the qualitative properties of the nonverbal actions, such as the amount of tension, strength, flow, shape, timing, and spatial focus. By following and expanding on the details of the young child's cues, the therapist creates a co-regulatory state, simultaneously sensing how the body actions and behaviors the patient and parents present provide clues about their feelings and the therapist's countertransference reactions. This is essential to build and maintain a secure and playful relationship, and is the key to establishing a sense of safety on emotional and neurophysiological levels.

Porges (2004, p. 19) established the term "neuroception" to describe the neural process in which we evaluate risk, frequently outside our own awareness, that can cause one to shift into a bodily state of defense, the

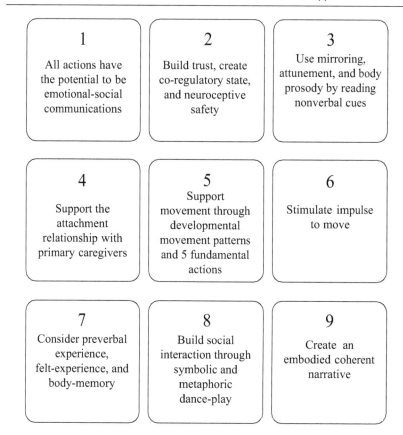

Figure 3.1 Medical DMT Intervention Strategies with Young Children with Medical Illness and Their Families

fight/flight mobilizing state, or, when sensing a severe threat to life, the immobilizing state of freezing or feigning death. In his case vignette of a child who, at age 4, underwent an 18-month treatment for leukemia, Porges discusses how the defensive mobilization state can compromise the ability to perceive positive social cues and create asocial behaviors, including aggression and withdrawal (Porges & Daniel, 2017). Facial cues, eye gaze, awareness of muscle tension, prosody of vocalizations and verbalizations, physical proximity, responses to different qualities of touch and "body prosody" – a term coined by Gray to describe how the dance therapist expands and improvises her body actions and gestures to "move the words" (Gray & Porges, 2017, p. 114) – are embodied tools, used by the dance therapist to develop trust. By animating actions and verbalizations during face-to-face interactions, while staying attuned to the patient's ability to receive input, the dance therapist creates playful attuned experiences that down-regulate defensive bodily reactions (Gray & Porges, 2017). As expressed by Gray and Porges, "Movement is a key to shifting physiological state. If you move, your autonomic state recruits sympathetic excitation, and when in a state of sympathetic excitation, the dorsal vagal pathways are inhabited and you *cannot* shut down" (2017, p. 112). With expressive movement as the primary tool, a dance therapist can shift the patient's emotional and physiological state in this unique way, building a rapport and facilitating therapeutic change.

The techniques of mirroring and attuning are used to dialogue verbally and nonverbally with the patient and caregivers (Tortora, 2006). Mirroring in DMT is an exact matching of affect and action, whereas in attunement, nonverbal qualities such as tone and mood of the mover's actions are responded to without exactly matching specific actions. The therapist uses these two techniques extensively and with extreme focus, carefully attending to the mover's reactions before adding or expanding her own actions.

Dance therapists also consider the neuromuscular developmental patterns a pediatric patient presents. Due to their illness and treatment side effects, young patients are at risk for delays or declines in functional mobility, loss of motoric milestones, and higher-level motor skills. Working from an integrated whole-child approach, the dance therapist observes how the young patient's developmental motor experience may be influencing her perceptions as they inform psychological development. The dance therapist is specifically attuned to the role interoception (our conscious and unconscious awareness of the sensations occurring in our body) plays in aligning internal sensations and actions with emotional feelings in the formation of an embodied self-identity (Erickson, 2021).

Here the motor and movement developmental work of Irmgard Bartenieff and Bonnie Bainbridge Cohen are useful. Bartenieff, a physical therapist, was one of the early dance therapists who introduced movement developmental sequences and a nonverbal analysis systematic vocabulary to the field in the United States (Bartenieff & Lewis, 1980; Levy, 2005). Cohen, an occupational therapist and first-generation protégée of Bartenieff, studies the neuromaturational developmental process of the infant's first year of life. Both colleagues use the term developmental movement patterns to reference how a baby acquires body coordination via the movement qualities of tension, strength, timing, and spatial orientation as the baby progresses through neuromotor skills. Bartenieff created a series of movement sequences, emphasizing particular body coordinations, to provide inner support and integrity based on one's experience of their body structure. Cohen arranged these six body coordinations in developmental order to emphasize their sequential prevalence: breath-flow, core-distal, head-tail, upper-lower, body-half, and contralateral body coordination. Cohen's work outlines the primary developmental movement patterns, the basic neurocellular patterns (BNP), describing them as the "underlying structural words or phrases of our movement" that influence our "physical, perceptual, emotional, and cognitive functioning" (Bainbridge Cohen, 2018, p. vi). A key element of Cohen's theoretical perspective is the correlation between the exploration of these developmental motor sequences via five fundamental actions associated with psychological phases of self-development (Erickson, 2021). These actions – yield, push, reach, grasp, and pull – provide dynamic ways for the baby to actively feel the impact of her moving body on her world. Each of these patterns act as a foundation for the next pattern, focusing baby's attention and engagement internally and progressing to external awareness through intentional interactions with the surroundings. It is through these embodied explorations that the baby's sense of body is engaged, contributing to the infant's sense of self and body-image formation. The baby's spatial experience of these motor patterns, progressing through the horizontal, sagittal, and vertical planes (this sequence is also described as horizontal, vertical, and sagittal by Bartenieff and others in the field), orients the baby's emotional, communicative, and interactive experience between self and other (Bainbridge Cohen, 2018; Bartenieff & Lewis, 1980; Eddy, 2016; Tortora, 2006). Table 3.1 provides

Table 3.1 Developmental Movement Patterns and Five Fundamental Actions

1. Basic vertebral movement patterns:
   a. Spinal – orientation of all limb patterns toward the midline, using movement of the spine.
   b. Homologous – symmetrical two-limb initiation patterns, integrating and differentiating upper and lower body, establishing broad-based support.
   c. Homolateral – asymmetrical one-limb initiating patterns, using upper and lower limbs on the same side; moving together or sequentially; establishing lateral line orientation by integrating left- and right-sidedness; belly crawling.
   d. Contralateral – asymmetrical one-limb initiating patterns using upper and lower limbs on opposite side; integrating diagonal use of limbs; orienting three-dimensionally; crawling on hands and knees.
2. Orienting body and movement to three spatial planes.
   a. Horizontal – created through horizontal and sagittal dimensions. Baby experiences rotation around vertical body axis, supporting rolling.
      i. *Psychophysical state:*"Communication plane" as baby takes in world from horizontal orientation, exploring front, sides, and back of body.
   b. Sagittal – created through sagittal and vertical dimensions. Experienced through flexion and extension, lifting head and spine up/away from supportive surface.
      i. *Psychophysical state:*"Here I come, there I go" plane, as baby mobilizes, approaches, and withdraws engagement, moving forward and backward.
   c. Vertical – created through vertical and horizontal dimensions. Experienced through lateral flexion on one side, while extending laterally on the other side. Flexion provides an experience of condensing, grounding, and strength, while elongation supports expansion, spaciousness, and lightness.
      i. *Psychophysical state:*"Here I am" plane, explore balance and control as baby moves up and down, and side to side.

3. Yield and push patterns:

   a. Ground body, developing strength through movements, providing sensation of condensing body within baby's kinespheric space (defined as one's personal space within one's reach), as baby yields into a supportive surface and then pushes against it.

   b. Psychophysical states:

      i. Supports internal awareness and intention.

      ii. *Yielding* creates sense of safety and trust as baby actively responds to gravity by increasing body tone, to rest or mobilize body while in contact, engaging with environment.

      iii. *Pushing* against a surface, baby differentiates self, sensing power, weight, internal support, body boundaries, and presence.

      iv. Inactive, flaccid response to gravity creates sense of heaviness, inertia, shutting off engagement within self and environment, as baby passively collapses into gravity.

4. Reach and pull patterns:

   a. Elongate the body creating lightness and mobility supporting spatial explorations.

   b. Psychophysical states:

      i. Orient baby's attention externally.

      ii. *Reaching* supports the baby's curiosity, orienting the baby to an object or person outside of self as the baby extends his body into space.

      iii. *Grasping* creates contact with an external object or person, creating a sense of accomplishment and strength when successfully obtaining and maintaining this contact.

      iv. *Pulling* brings an object or person closer to the baby, solidifying a sense of accomplishment and connection between self and other.

      v. Motor sequences involving *reaching, grasping,* and *pulling* support urge to take action, spontaneously extending beyond self to engage with others and surroundings.

      vi. Difficulty with these actions can manifest in dampening desire and an outer intention to respond to the environment.

Note: Data from Tortora (2006); Eddy (2016); Bainbridge Cohen (2018)

an outline of the developmental movement patterns and the five fundamental actions with their psychological associations.

In dance/movement therapy, we look at how the child's experience of motor and developmental movement patterns influences their perceptions and emotional development (see Tortora, 2006, for an in-depth discussion). Though a complete description goes beyond the focus of this book, the basic principles most relevant to the dance therapist's work include how the infant's medical condition and treatment impact her ability to experience these sequences, with their corresponding action-based psychological expression. Using the BNP and five fundamental actions as guidelines, sessions include:

- Orienting the baby's body and movement in relationship with the three spatial planes and six coordinations: breath-flow, core-distal, head-tail, upper-lower, body-half, contralateral.
- Exploring the initiation and sequencing of basic vertebrate-movement patterns through the body.

- Exploring how the five fundamental actions (yield, push, reach, grasp, and pull) inform the baby's emotional/social experience, and how they offer movement-based opportunities to use these actions to create embodied self-agency.

When working with this very young, medically ill population, we must consider how the infant's experiences of movement restrictions – including frequent supine and side-lying positioning, and decreased opportunities to physically explore the environment to support postural control, balance, and transitions between postures – impact their natural curiosity for movement explorations, emotional experience, and overall mental health. For example, how might an infant who is not able to reach, grasp, and pull as protective responses internalize this experience? When this happens over time, how might the infant's basic trust and security be compromised on a deeply embodied level? These questions are exemplified in the following vignette.

Carla, diagnosed with acute myeloid leukemia (AML) at 9.5 months, has spent most of her life in the hospital. She has endured several surgeries and, due to the metiport on her chest, spends most of her time lying on her back. Her parents split their time with her so that she is always with one of them. They are warm, loving, and attentive to her. Carla is breastfed and often in her mom's arms when I arrive for our dance therapy session.

Though Carla receives physical and occupational therapy regularly, she is not able to sit up independently in her crib and does not reach for toys presented to her, both tasks that are expected developmentally at her age. Sitting up on Mom's lap for support, Carla is alert and curious, watching as I drape a colorful silk scarf across her feet. Though attentive, she does not reach for the scarf. Mom, always quick to anticipate Carla's needs, instinctively reaches to lift it into Carla's hands, which are resting on Mom's legs. I smile at Mom, silently motioning for her to pause as I put on a Bob Marley reggae song – one of Carla and Mom's favorites. I want to see if the laid-back rhythmic flow might encourage Carla to initiate her own reaching actions. Upon hearing the music, Carla smiles and instantly rocks her own body to the beat. Mom and I pick up both ends of the colorful scarf and flutter it toward and away from Carla's reach. She tracks the action with her eyes and lifts up her arm. We let the scarf linger closer to her body, within her near-reach space, and she grasps the soft silk. As she holds on, in tune with the rhythm, we all gently rock forward and backward. Caught up in our dancing flow, Carla inevitably loses her grasp of the scarf. This time she shifts her body forward and reaches her arm out much farther, catching the scarf as we dance it to-and-fro. Her exuberant giggle and her increasingly excited actions radiate her pride in her successful grasp, topped only by Mom's enthusiastic responses.

As we continue this dancing game, Carla's reach continues to extend, and her playful mood endures. At our next session, Mom demonstrates with much satisfaction all the ways she and Carla have played this dance-game, and how much stronger, more physically explorative and playful Carla has become.

Clinical Discussion

Carla's initial behaviors raise the question of whether she has a neurological or medically induced deficit, or if she has not had enough opportunity to initiate movement because Mom has a pattern of anticipating Carla's needs. The power of Tortora's nonverbal intervention shows how quickly Carla can physically engage when she is given time and space. Typically, it is very difficult for any parent to tolerate their baby's distress; it is even more difficult when a child is ill. It is instinctive for parents to do even the simplest things for them. Though it may seem very subtle, helping Mom pause to give Carla the chance to successfully reach for the scarf on her own provides Carla with a much-needed physical sense of agency, which Mom immediately understands and builds on during her own play with her baby. This nuanced intervention made a change at the representational level to Mom's perception of her child's strengths and weaknesses. Such a change in perspective occurs over time, as Tortora continues to guide and support Carla's parents to play this way, encouraging the parents to pause to read Carla's nonverbal cues and give Carla extra time to respond. This type of engagement happens through repeated interactions; it is not a one-time intervention.

Movement as the Bridge in the Use of Imagination and Pretend Play

Building on the felt experience of primary movement patterns in infancy, the dance therapist pays keen attention to the symbolic implications of the body experience and the images, story themes, and pretend play in which the child engages. Chodorow (1991, p. 12), a dance therapist and Jungian analyst, states: "Dance and pretend . . . [are] synonymous." This aptly portrays the dance therapist's use of dance as an elaboration of pretend play that enables the patient to engage in symbolic expression. As discussed in Chapter 2, language understanding evolves from our minds simulating our physical experiences. Prior to linguistic expression, it is our corporality, of which our bodies are the source, which shapes our conceptual understandings. In his paper about the role of metaphor and imagination in child development, Haen (2020), a drama and creative arts therapist specializing in trauma work with youth and families, discusses how pretend play, first initiated by caregivers during infancy, is a significant component of the attachment relationship that builds engagement and co-regulation. He states that by

12 months, infants show the ability to engage in symbolism and fantasy play. During the second year of life, and more prominent in 3–5-year-olds, the child initiates pretend play. Haen's description of the therapeutic use of metaphor and imagination in play matches the dance therapist's perspective: He describes this as a tool that increases the child's sense of agency and mastery over difficult and/or traumatic experiences and memories. This play recontextualizes the experiences, reorganizing them into a new perspective.

This is illustrated in the vignette in Chapter 2, describing a group session with Maor, that occurred prior to a treatment he was quite anxious about. Maor becomes an army general, organizing his "soldiers" – the therapists and his parents – in marching order through the unpredictable vastitudes of a battle. Following his commands, we use a silk scarf to create a rainbow after combat, culminating in a beautiful scene whereby Maor assists us in rocking a baby doll in the scarf as Mom sings a lullaby. Taking the stance of the general, Maor experiences his need for agency in the face of the overwhelming aspects of his medical treatment and his need for nurturance within the loving embrace of his caregivers, enacted through the baby doll and Mom's spontaneous singing. When working with toddlers and early elementary-age patients, the dance therapist provides dance-play activities that enable the expression, symbolic examination, and reflection of the child's current experience, contributing to the development of an embodied coherent narrative of the overall medical experience.

Props, Tools, and Techniques

As is evident in the vignettes throughout this book, the dance therapist uses a variety of props and tools to help the child "tell their story." For infants and babies, these props are primarily sensorial, engaging the infant's embodiment experience, supporting regulation, and stimulating development. Our bodies and actions – the therapist's and the child's – are the central communicative and healing tools with musical instruments, recorded music, and props like colorful, sheer scarves, balls, and bubbles stimulating additional sensory engagement. For toddlers, props are added to support the child's more active involvement in physical and emotional regulation, and to offer more sensitively approached representational enactments. Tools that teach the child how to become aware of their own body–mind–emotional continuum to enhance regulation occur through activities such as embodying different energy speeds the child's body state presents using a four-colored "Speed Spiral" chart: Different emotional states and thoughts are mapped to these speeds, identified by using feeling charts and books about emotions. Erica Willheim (2021, p. 45), a clinical psychologist specializing in trauma play therapy, has created a useful categorization of props for children ages 3–12, which specially supports a "bottom-up" neurosequential model to create "patterned, repetitive, rhythmic somatosensory activities." These props, which are also commonly used in DMT, include resistive materials for sensory play, such as cocooning Lycra fabric, clay, tug-of-war with bungee cords, and material to build play tents; regulation games such as Simon Says and Red Light/Green light; props that enable expansive body movement and physical re-enactments; and tools for body regulation, such as fidgets and other hand manipulatives, squishy and bumpy sensory balls, and weighted vests or blankets. DMT sessions can also include classic play therapy props such as dolls, dollhouses, and other doll-play materials, books, pretend food, role-play and dress-up dance costumes, and those that evoke the trauma experience, such as ambulances and medical toy props. Typically, in DMT, these props are used to augment the storied themes of the characters embodied by the child and therapist. They can also be used to create distance from traumatic themes and lower arousal if there is concern that full-body enactment could be triggering. A full list of these props is outlined in Chapter 12.

Structure of a DMT Session in a Private Clinic and Pediatric Setting: SPEED 3R

In the private clinical setting, the body–mind–emotional continuum activities previously described, designed to enhance regulation, usually occur as "warm-up" activities at the start of the session. They are a precursor to the central part of the session when children choose props that evoke enactment stories, enabling an embodied reprocessing of their experiences by supporting different, more empowering solutions and endings to the stories they create. *Carefully* supported active dance-play re-enactments provide a primary processing of medical experiences that support healing due to the body–mind–emotional integration this full-body exploration enables. The word *carefully* is italicized to highlight that in DMT, enactment dance-plays provide a means of remembering difficult events rather than creating a reliving of these potentially traumatic memories that may be present on a body-sensation level, instead of a cognizant awareness on the young child's part. Sessions typically end with a drawing, writing, and retelling of the story, and a "cool down" involving breath awareness, progressive relaxation, and other calming multisensory activities (Tortora & Whitley, 2019). The creative physical actions of this ending have a body and emotional regulatory function as the child experiencing containment and closure in the dance-play story. During treatment, these sessions occur in varying combinations, depending on the pressing emotional needs of the child and their parents. They include individual sessions with the child and therapist, sessions with the child and caregivers, and individual sessions with the therapist and parents.

In the medical setting, sessions can be individual, with caregivers, or in groups, and can include other medical staff such as nurses and doctors. Sessions occur at bedside, inpatient, outpatient, or even in the waiting room. Sessions begin by following the patient's lead, with the child obviously initiating the session; or by the therapist observing the child's present behaviors and arousal state and initiating activities while staying sensitively attuned, enabling the child's responses to then direct the progression of the session. One day, the child may present himself in a very tired, listless mood, needing soothing, quiet engagement – and the next day, he may be sitting up, eager to get out of bed to dance around the room. Improvisation, a prominent modern dance method, is especially useful training for dance therapists because the patient's state and condition can change rapidly and unexpectedly even within a session. By accommodating to any mood the patient presents, the dance therapist builds therapeutic rapport, while supporting the child's felt experience to gain control over some aspects of their medical treatment.

While observing the patient's present physical and emotional state, the dance therapist keeps the following questions in mind throughout the session:

1. How does the patient's unique way of relating and moving reflect the patient's experience of his/her illness?
2. How does the patient's experience of their illness color his/her unique way of relating and moving?
3. What does it feel like to experience the world through that patient's particular expressive movement repertoire?
4. How can a therapeutic environment be structured to enable the patient to experience his/her nonverbal expression as a communicative tool, while simultaneously enabling the patient, to use that experience to explore new ways of coping with his/her illness?

(Tortora, 2015a, p. 172)

These questions enable the dance therapist to decipher the underlying personality of the young patient to create session activities to support coping and enable the patient to experience himself beyond the restrictions of his illness.

The acronym SPEED 3R (Table 3.2) summarizes the core components of the session.

Table 3.2 Core Components of DMT Hospital Session: SPEED 3R

S ocializing
P lay
E xercise
E mpowerment through expression
D ancing – joyful creativity, healing

R elease
R ecuperation
R esilience – from invasive medical treatment experience

Socializing supports the young patient's growing capacity to engage with others, which is especially important during early stages of development because increased stranger anxiety and avoidance can manifest easily when so many medical staff are engaged in the patient's care.

Play is a natural way that children explore their feelings and is an essential developmental skill. The use of fantasy and imaginary play is the primary way a child processes the world around her (Winnicott, 1982). It is also very helpful for caregivers to see their child playfully engaging in the midst of her medical care. The classic Piagetian principle (Piaget, 1962) that babies first learn through sensory-motor experience supports the movement and multisensory activities and props used in DMT (Vincent et al., 2007).

Exercise – moving one's body naturally – enables the patient to engage in spontaneous and structured activities. The physicality of DMT can also support physical and occupational therapy goals. Dance therapists are invited to co-treat with these therapists, bringing a playful expressive focus to the skills being worked on.

Empowerment, as discussed throughout this book, results from the focus of all DMT activities on the belief that being able to engage in emotionally expressive body and movement-based activities is strengthening. Enabling the patient to direct the activities provides an embodied sense of mastery, competence, and autonomy, which is especially powerful during a time when many of the medical treatment protocols do not allow for this.

Dancing, with its inherent healing properties, provides a means of creative and aesthetic personal and group expression without words, which can shift the intensity of the situation.

The last three Rs of the acronym summarize the overall goals of the DMT experience: Releasing feelings in the moment supports Recuperation and builds Resilience to be able to cope throughout the medical experience. With this youngest population, common behavioral reactions to acute stress include a sense of powerlessness; withdrawal, disengagement, defensive self-protective behaviors; and emotional, social, physical, cognitive, and communicative regression to an earlier developmental stage, such as a resurgence of stranger anxiety. This can be compounded by the caregiver's own sense of helplessness, suffering, and guilt. But these last three Rs support growth vs. regression. DMT sessions conducted over the full course of treatment create opportunities to develop strong relationships that support the patient and family members in their immediate and long-term needs.

Conclusion

Our responses to a baby's nonverbal communications can empower even the youngest patients as they experience their expressive actions resulting in attuned responses from adults. We don't have to wait until infants have verbal skills to enable them to feel they are good communicators. Providing young patients with a way to explore their experience can create a sense of agency during their treatment and an embodied coherent narrative of their experience. Helping parents read their baby's cues also gives them a sense of agency as they continue to build the ability to care for their child during stressful times. Pediatric DMT is uniquely positioned to support the healthy development of very young children and empower their families to more successfully navigate the emotional challenges of the medical experience.

References

ADTA (2021). Retrieved March 29, 2021 from https://adta.memberclicks.net/what-is-dancemovement-therapy

Bainbridge Cohen, B. (2018). *Basic neurocellular patterns: Exploring developmental movement*. Burchfield Rose Publishers.

Bartenieff, I., & Lewis, D. (1980). *Body movements: Coping with the environment*. Gordon and Breach Science Publishers.

Bernstein, P. (1979). *Eight theoretical approaches in dance – movement therapy*. Kendall/Hunt Publishing Company.

Bloom, K. (2006). *The embodied self: Movement and psychoanalysis*. Karnac.

Chodorow, J. (1991). *Dance therapy and depth psychology: The moving imagination*. Routledge.

Cloitre, M., Stolbach, B., Herman, J., van de Kolk, B., Pynoos, R., Want, J., & Petkova, E. (2009). A developmental approach to complex PTSD: Childhood and adult cumulative trauma as predictors of symptom complexity. *Journal of Traumatic Stress*, 22(5), 399–408.

Cohen, S. O. (1996). Before the stillness-dance therapy helps the young communicate before they die. *Hospice Magazine*.

Cohen, S. O. (1999, November–December). Dance/movement therapy: How it's helping cancer survivors coping. *Coping*.

Cohen, S. O. (2000, Fall). Integrating dance/movement therapy principles into child life practice. *Child Life Focus*, 2(2).

Cohen, S. O., & Walco, G. (1999). Dance/movement therapy for children and adolescents with cancer. *Cancer Practice*, 7(1), 34–42.

Eddy, M. (2016). *Mindful movement: The evolution of the somatic arts and conscious action*. Intellect, The University of Chicago Press.

Erickson, L. (2021). Sensing the body: A dance/movement therapy model of embodied identity development. *Body, Movement and Dance in Psychotherapy*, 16(3), 202–217. https://doi.org/10.1080/17432979.2020.1850524

Goodill, S. (2005). *An introduction to medical dance/movement therapy*. Jessica Kingsley Publishers.

Goodill, S. (2018). Accumulating evidence for dance/movement therapy in cancer care. *Frontiers in Psychology*, 9(1778). https://doi.org/10.3389/fpsyg.2018.01778

Goodill, S., & Morningstar, D. (1993). The role of dance/movement therapy with medically ill children. *International Journal of Arts Medicine*, 2, 24–27.

Gray, A. E., & Porges, S. W. (2017). Polyvagal-informed dance/movement therapy with children who shut down: Restoring core rhythmicity. In C. Malchiodo & D. Crenshaw (Eds.), *What to do when children clam up in psychotherapy* (pp. 102–136). Guilford Press.

Haen, C. (2020, 2020/01/02). The roles of metaphor and imagination in child trauma treatment. *Journal of Infant, Child, and Adolescent Psychotherapy*, 19(1), 42–55. https://doi.org/10.1080/15289168.2020.1717171

Hervey, L. W. (2007). Embodied ethical decision making. *American Journal of Dance Therapy*, 29(2), 91–108. https://doi.org/10.1007/s10465-007-9036-5

Koch, S., & Fischman, D. (2011). Embodied enactive dance/movement therapy. *American Journal of Dance Therapy*, 33, 57–32.

Koch, S., Kunz, T., Lykou, S., & Cruz, R. (2014). Effects of dance movement therapy and dance on psychological outcomes: A meta-analysis. *The Arts in Psychotherapy*, 41(1), 46–64.

Levine, P. (2012). *In an unspoken voice: How the body releases trauma*. North Atlantic Books.

Levine, P., & Kline, M. (2008). *Trauma-proofing your kids: A parent's guide for instilling confidence, joy and resilience*. North Atlantic Books.

Levy, F. (1995). *Dance and other expressive art therapies: When words are not enough*. Routledge.

Levy, F. (2005). *Dance movement therapy: A healing art revised edition* (Rev. ed.). American Alliance for Health, Physical Education, Recreation and Dance.

Madden, J., Mowry, P., Gao, D., Cullen, P., & Foreman, N. (2010). Creative arts therapy improves quality of life for pediatric brain tumor patients receiving outpatient chemotherapy. *Journal of Pediatric Oncology Nursing*, 27(3), 133–145. https://doi.org/10:1177/1043454209355452

Mendelsohn, J. (1999). Dance/movement therapy with hospitalized children. *American Journal of Dance Movement Therapy*, 21(2), 65–80.

Minde, K. (2000). Prematurilty and serious medical conditions in infancy: Implications for development, behavior, and intervention In C. Zeanah (Ed.), *Handbook of infant mental health* (2nd ed., pp. 176–194). The Guildford Press.

Nir, Y. (1985). Post-truamatic stress disorder in children with cancer. In S. Eth & R. Pynoos (Eds.), *Post-truamatic stress disorder in children* (pp. 123–132). American Psychatric Association Publishing.

Pallaro, P. (Ed.). (1999). *Authentic movement: Essays by mary starks whitehouse, janet adler and joan chodorow*. Jessica Kingsley Press.

Piaget, J. (1962). *Play, dreams and imitation in childhood*. Norton.

Porges, S. W. (2004). Neuroception: A subconcious system for detecting threats and safety. *Zero to Three*, 24(5), 19–24.

Porges, S. W., & Daniel, S. (2017). Play and dynamics of treating pediatric medical trauma. In S. Daniel & C. Trevarthen (Eds.), *Rhythms of relating in children's therapies: Connecting creatively with vunerable children* (pp. 113–124). Jessica Kingsley Publishers.

Roberts, M. (2021). Embodied ethical decision-making: A clinical case study of respect for culturally based meaning making in mental healthcare. *American Journal of Dance Therapy*, 43(1), 36–63. https://doi.org/10.1007/s10465-020-09338-3

Schechter, D. S. (2017). Traumatically skewed intersubjectivity. *Psychoanalytic Inquiry*, 37(4), 251–264. https://doi.org/10:1080/07351690.2017.1299500

Terr, L. (1992). *Too scared to cry: How trauma affects children . . . and untimately us all*. Basic Books.

Tortora, S. (2006). *The dancing dialogue: Using the communicative power of movement with young children*. Paul H. Brookes Publishing Company.

Tortora, S. (2015a). Dance/movement psychotherapy in early childhood treatment and pediatric oncology. In S. Chaiklin & H. Wengrower (Eds.), *The art and science of dance/movement therapy: Life is dance*. Routledge.

Tortora, S. (2015b). Mindfulness and movement. In C. S. Willard (Ed.), *Teaching mindfulness skills to kids and teens*. Guildford Press.

Tortora, S. (2016, October 6–7). *Dance/movement therapy in psycho-oncology: Are there evidences of its efficacy?* Proceedings of the Complimentary Therapies in Oncology: Dance, Yoga, Music, Art, Brescia, Italy.

Tortora, S. (2019). Children are born to dance! Pediatric medical dance/movement therapy: The view from integrative pediatric oncology. *Children*, 6(14), 1–27. https://doi.org/10.3390/children6010014

Tortora, S., & Whitley, J. (2019). Mother-son transgenerational transmission of eating issues using a co-treatment method. In H. Payne, S. Koch, J. Tantia, & T. Fuchs (Eds.), *International handbook of embodied perspectives in psychotherapy: Approaches from dance movement, the arts and body psychotherapies*. Routledge Publishers.

van der Kolk, B. (2015). *The body keeps the score: Brain, mind and body in the healing of trauma*. Penguin Books.

Vincent, S. R., Tortora, S., Shaw, J., Basiner, J., Devereaux, C., Mulcahy, S., & Ponsini, M. (2007). Collaborating with a mission: The Andréa Rizzo Foundation spreads the gift of dance/movement therapy. *American Journal of Dance Therapy*, 29(1), 51–58.

Willheim, E. (2021). Presentation to ways of seeing international training program, Online Training.

Winnicott, D. W. (1982). *Playing and reality*. Tavistock Publications.

Zilius, M. (2010). Dance movement therapy in pediatrics: An overview. *Alternative & Complimentary Therapies: A New Bimonthly Publication for Health Care Practitioners*, 16(2), 87–92.

Chapter 4

Affect and Self-Regulation in Social and Emotional Development

Introduction

This chapter focuses on the impact of medical illness on the infant's ability to learn self-regulation, encompassing both emotion and physiological regulation. A child's self-regulatory skill greatly impacts her social and emotional behavior. Being able to regulate emotion and physiological input during early childhood can set the template for later psychological, physical, cognitive, social, behavioral, and academic styles of organization and well-being. At birth, the newborn's capacity for self-regulation is limited (Zeanah, 2019), but during the infant's first few months and year, the complexity of her emotional life expands as she gains the ability to initiate and engage emotionally and respond to the emotional expressions of others.

A systematic review of 28 studies from 1990–2019 examining the psychosocial outcomes of infants and young children – from birth to 6 years, 11 months old – with congenital heart disease (CHC) found that "young children are at risk of impaired emotional, social, and behavioral development, and importantly, that symptoms of psychosocial impairment are detectable very early in infancy" (Clancy et al., 2019, p. 13). They cite robust research with school-age children that demonstrates heightened risk for neurodevelopmental impairment, including lower cognitive scores, fine and gross motor difficulties, and adaptive behavior problems, compared with typically developing peers. Research predicting social functioning in children ages 1.5–5 years with cochlear implants found similar issues with emotion regulation and social functioning when compared with typically developing hearing children (Wiefferink et al., 2012). Children with cochlear implants had less adequate emotion-regulation strategies and less social competence in contrast to their peers, whose social competence was not related to emotion regulation.

The relationship between emotion and physiological regulation within the often foreign, invasive, and multisensory stimuli and arduous treatments that a young child with a medical illness must process adds a layer of complexity that needs focused attention to best support these infants

DOI: 10.4324/9781003134800-5

and their parents. Presenting an in-depth explanation of each theory goes beyond the scope of this book, but it is sufficient to say that most literature concerning social and emotional development agrees that self-regulation – and more specifically, emotion and physiological regulation – occurs within the context of social relationships.

This chapter includes a review of the research on and understanding of typical self-regulation and emotion regulation, and the foundational role early social relationships play in these developments in infancy and early childhood within the context to young children with medical illness. The chapter concludes with an introduction to the Embodied Parenting program, developed by Tortora. Embodied Parenting teaches parents how to reflect on and attune to their infant's and their own nonverbal cues to support self-regulation and co-regulation, and to enhance and strengthen their attachment relationship.

Affect Regulation and Attachment Security in Young Children with Medical Illness

There is a link between attachment security and affect regulation that becomes apparent when observing the dynamics of the parent–infant relationship involving a young child with a medical illness. Within the parent–infant relationship is the core component of attachment: The way the infant represents his caregiver's protective is considered a significant feature in creating a safe holding environment. Bowlby (1969) theorized that babies are biologically disposed to look for an attachment figure while they are in distress, and to explore their environment from their secure base. Optimally, the two systems are in balanced interplay; whenever the child is in distress, the attachment system is activated and the exploratory one is deactivated. Parents vary in their ability to provide protection and comfort in times of perceived danger. A secure base, or safe haven, functions as the key ingredient in a relationship that provides emotional and physiological regulation and has been linked to the development of empathy and mentalization skills later in development.

This is very relevant in extremely stressful situations when an infant is diagnosed with a serious and/or potentially life-threatening condition, when the parent's own attachment system is activated by stress. Secure attachment is a protective factor for the parent and infant to cope with illness-related difficulties. The outcome for the child in very adverse situations is the result of a complex interplay between risk and protective factors in the infant, caregivers, and their environment (Sameroff & MacKenzie, 2003). The parents' ability to provide a strong, consistent, safe, holding environment throughout the medical experience can boost their sense of successful parenting. However, the emotional pain and strife of *not* being able to protect their baby from illness and the ensuing treatments can greatly impact the parents' confidence in their relationship with their child. The infant's own characteristics also greatly impact how he reacts to illness. The medical experience deeply affects the whole family, leaving lasting impressions that can surface later in attitudes and behaviors, which may at first appear unrelated to the early medical experience. For example, the child may become overly agitated when not feeling in control of her environment, quick to tantrum, or avoidant of touch, even when parents provide loving touch. And the parents may be overly protective or fearful of setting limits, which is unconsciously informed by worry about upsetting the child.

The infant's temperament is a very important variable, as Woodhouse and colleagues have shown in their research about maternal responses to irritable babies (Cassidy et al., 2005). The specific maternal behaviors examined are the mother's availability to calm the baby during times of distress, when crying, not fussing, by soothing the infant through chest-to-chest holding until the infant is completely calm, picking up the infant when he strongly signals this desire, and not presenting responses that frighten the infant (Woodhouse et al., 2019). Behaviors that promote a calm regulatory state during infant explorations include the ability to support calm connectedness; repair moments that interrupt the infant's capability to stay calmly regulated without terminating exploration; being available for eye contact when the infant is seeking social connection, while not soliciting eye contact that usurps the infant's capacity to set the pace; and sharing in delight when initiated by the infant. These behaviors demonstrate the caregiver's ability to read and anticipate the baby's cues to prevent stress and dysregulation when the baby is susceptible to becoming upset. Through these caregiving behaviors, the infant learns she can trust her parent to provide a safe, secure base.

Supporting parents of babies with medical illness to use these specific nonverbal caregiver behaviors during times of distress, throughout and after medical care, has the potential to ease the baby's and the parent's experience and support their relationship.

Self-Regulation in Early Infancy

Early regulatory capacities have long-lasting impact on a child's functioning. Barlow and colleagues reference the research of DeGangi et al. (2000), who state that 95 percent of infants age 7 months who had moderate regulatory difficulties in areas such as "sleep and feeding; ability to self-soothe and modulate affect states; ability to regulate mood, and emotional and [behavioral] control" were experiencing relationship problems in primary relationships at age three (Barlow et al., 2018, p. 7). The caregiver's ability to understand and respond appropriately to the baby's temperament, as it determines her style of engaging in the world, influences the baby's social, emotional, cognitive, and behavioral development, ultimately mediating health issues along the life span. Hofer, who created the term "hidden regulators," was the first researcher to describe the underlying neuropsychophysiological basis for this:

> It is likely that during the early mother-infant relationship in humans, these hidden regulatory interactions come to be experienced by the infant as synchrony, reciprocity, and warmth, or as dissonance and frustration, depending on variations in their timing, contiguity, or patterning. With the maturation of learning and memory, the traces of these early regulatory interactions are organized into mental representations and emotional states thought to constitute the "internal working model" of attachment theory . . . . They promise to afford a bridge between biology and psychology in the study of early development and of social relationships later in life.
>
> (Hofer, 1995, p. 204)

Hofer's research reveals that the mother's – that is, the primary caregiver's – behavioral actions affect the infant in biological and behavioral domains of development, both as they emerge and in the long term. Examining how infants acquire self-regulatory skills offers a road map for looking at child development through the lens of developing coping strategies for parents caring for a young child with a medical illness.

For an infant with a medical illness, the stress threshold and pursuit of self-regulation can be challenging, or even be compromised beyond the early months of life. Invasive procedures, surgeries, life-sustaining equipment, and daily medically oriented physical handling occurs disproportionately, creating stressors to which these babies must learn to adapt and regulate as part of their embodied experience. If we take a closer look at state regulation, one of the most basic and important self-regulatory systems, we can see how regulation influences the pediatric patient's emotional expression of their embodied experience.

State regulation typically relates to the infant's ability to organize sleep and wake and crying cycles in relation to input/output stimuli as portrayed through observable nonverbal behaviors. Wolff (1987) is one of the original early-infancy researchers to use individual motor coordination and movement patterns as the features of behavioral states in self-organization, with an emphasis on wakefulness. Wolff emphasizes that as infants acquire increased sensorimotor, postural control, and behavior-state coordination, they are less dependent on, sensitive to, and disrupted by environmental stimuli. As infant behavior states shift into more voluntary, self-initiated control, and are mutually interactive, they create more internal stability during wakefulness. Wolff's focus on studying motor patterns associated with these states and distinguishing between behavior as an expression of emotions or as a behavioral state is especially helpful in working with infants with a medical illness. These infants must work hard to maintain or regain state regulation that can be disrupted by medical procedures. Learning how to "read" the infant's unique style or nonverbal expression of emotion within the context of achieving behavior regulation is essential to best support the infant's biopsychosocial needs and assess how the infant's behaviors impact parents and other significant caregivers.

Emotion Regulation

Emotion regulation (ER) is considered a core factor in a child's achievement of social-emotional competence (Calkins & Hill, 2006). Early childhood clinical referrals often occur because parents and day care or preschool teachers are concerned about a child's emotional dysregulation. Children who show emotion and behavior regulation demonstrate more flexible, spontaneous responses to situational changes in environment and are able to delay their responses when needed (Zeanah, 2019). Understanding the mechanisms that influence how our emotions evolve over time provides context for the embodied approach used in this book.

When used as a general term, ER is attached to a variety of definitions from a biological or psychological stance. All definitions include some level of organization and patterning of emotions to create a state of homeostasis on a physiological systems level and on a psychological level. ER includes the shaping of a rising emotion, and when it emerges, how it is experienced and expressed (Gross, 2013a). Gross states that ER is a component of emotional activation, rather than a response to it, and that it can contribute to maladaptive behaviors in adverse environmental conditions. Gross also asserts that an essential feature of ER is the activation of a goal to up-regulate or down-regulate the intensity or duration of an emotional response. From a neuroscientific view, throughout the infant and young child's early years, developmental neural mechanisms of regulation, cognition, and emotion are linked dynamically, contributing to how the child processes information and takes action to regulate emotion (Zeanah, 2019). ER can be intrinsic, activated within one's self, or extrinsic and interpersonal, activated in someone else, as exemplified when a parent tries to appear calm while soothing their child, when internally he is frightened by his child's diagnosis (Gross, 2013b).

Intrinsic features for infants include specific neural and physiological systems that are engaged during events that activate emotion control. Temperament is the main intrinsic feature influencing the development of emotion regulation. Although temperament is construed in multiple ways (Bates & Pettit, 2015; Carey & Me Devitt, 1978; Chess & Thomas, 1997; Rothbart et al., 2011; Shiner et al., 2012), in infancy it is consensually defined as constitutionally based biological, individual differences in attentional, motor, and emotional reactivity and self-regulation, which are exhibited in different contexts in response to stimulation (Chen & Schmidt, 2015; Rothbart, 2011). Perhaps the most widely adopted parent-report infant-temperament measure is the Infant Behavior Questionnaire (IBQ). Developed by Rothbart (1981, 2011), the IBQ consists of 94 items across six levels:

Activity: Gross motor activity.
Smiling and Laughter: Positive arousal under relatively quiet conditions.
Fear, Distress, and/or Extended Latency: To approach a novel stimulus.
Distress to Limitations: Reactions to frustrating conditions.
Duration of Orienting: Sustained attention when there is no change in stimulation.
Soothability: Reduction of fussing, crying, or distress to calming.

Factor analyses of the IBQ have yielded overarching factors related to positive and negative reactivity. Reactivity is measured by observing the infant's quickness in responding to an unfamiliar stressor, the intensity of the response, and the length of time it takes for the infant to recover. Contextualist models focus on the roles of environment and experience in the formation and expression of temperament, which is now understood to be open to exogenous influences (Rothbart, 2011). Higher levels of sensitive, warm parenting predict decreased negative reactivity in a child, even controlling for initial levels (Bates et al., 2012), and higher levels of harsh control predict increased negative reactivity, even controlling for initial levels (Braungart-Rieker et al., 2010). Low parental sensitive responsiveness predicts increased fear, controlling for initial levels (Pauli-Pott et al., 2004), and the inverse (Park et al., 1997). Thus, one might expect a changing temperament due to maturation of self-regulation and experience.

Observing and learning the individual differences in emotion reactivity in very young pediatric patients through their nonverbal cues can offer clues to providing more personally directed sensitive care during medical procedures. Being aware and attentive to these behaviors by pausing and pacing a procedure to allow for a moment of adjustment and loving care by a caregiver or nurse can redirect the infant's attention. This can provide a supportive felt experience that, if consistently followed as a course of treatment, will accumulate and help build the infant's embodied experience in developing later regulatory strategies and skills.

Orienting in Early Self-Regulation

Orienting and state regulation play key roles in modulating positive and negative affect and predict less distress in toddlerhood. Being able to look away during frightening or stressful events facilitates self-regulation of negative emotions. Alerting, orienting, and executive attention are the three neural-attention networks instrumental in self-regulation. Orienting is especially dominant at the beginning of life and significant in state regulation. In infancy, regulatory control of emotions and behavior begins in the brain's orienting network, shifting to the brain's executive network by age 3 or 4, when orienting takes on a secondary role to executive control.

Infants, early in life, naturally orient toward novelty; alerting and orienting networks support the achievement and sustenance of an alert state directed toward sensory stimuli. Before 3–4 months, infants have little control over orienting and go through a period of "obligatory attention," when they are unable to visually disengage from stimulus, even if this extended orienting causes distress (Rothbart et al., 2011, p. 208). Rothbart and her colleagues (2011) report that by four months, infants achieve some orienting control and can disengage, redirecting their attention to another location. Parent-reported measures of temperament associate this increased flexibility with the idea that infants having lower negative emotions and more soothability. Obligatory attention is an important behavior to keep in mind when performing medical procedures on infants of this age, because it can be misinterpreted as interest, attention, or compliance rather than distress.

Effortful control first appears in toddlerhood and preschool-age children. In infancy, showing caution by fixation before moving and fearfulness, demonstrated by the infant's reactive inhibition to novelty, is predictive of later effortful control. By 18–20 months, early signs of effortful control are evident in a decrease of surgency/positive control, interpreted as demonstrating the development of voluntary control of positive impulsivity. The data suggests that genetic makeup and parenting styles influence the transference from orienting to executive control network functioning (Rothbart et al., 2011), and this shift provides an avenue toward stronger self-regulation.

Role of Caregiving in Developing Self-Regulation

A large part of how well an infant's emotion regulation emerges in the earliest months is due to extrinsic supportive interactions with parents and other primary caregivers. During this time, parents are instrumental in helping infants learn how to redirect their attention. By 3–6 months, babies can be soothed from overstimulation distress by being presented with novel objects, such as visual and auditory stimulation, suggesting that the orienting network is active in emotional control early in life. In Western societies, caregivers increasingly use orienting with older infants when over-aroused (Rothbart et al., 2011). Research with 15-month-old infants shows that maternal sensitivity, mindfulness, and support of autonomy relate to the child's later executive functioning and self-regulatory activities at 18–20 months.

These findings all point to the important role the sensitive caregiver has in shaping a young child's behaviors, providing impetus for the baby's development of self-regulation by redirecting their attention to soothe during distress. Through the aid of a sensitive caregiver, the infant's natural propensity to orient attention toward novelty can also be used for soothing. By orienting the infant's attention away, the caregiver acts as a bridge, offering the infant an embodied experience of redirecting her attention. Exercising the orienting network supports connectivity with the later development of the executive network.

In the following vignette, Tortora has a DMT session with 6-month-old Brian, who at that time had been in the hospital for three months. Tortora demonstrates how she is able to sensitively reorient the baby's attention, supporting Brian's self-regulatory efforts through embodied sensing.

When I enter the room for my first dance/movement therapy session with Brian, he is in the arms of a hospital caregiver who is rocking him and attempting to direct his attention to a cartoon on the television. I observe Brian's nonverbal cues: His body is erect, and he holds himself apart from the caregiver's shoulder, looking away while crying. His cry is contained yet deep, causing his whole body to vibrate.

Brian is often without family present because his single mom has three other children at home to care for. As the caregiver gives Brian to me, she says he has been crying like this for the last 20 minutes and has not responded to her efforts to soothe him by holding and rocking him.

First, I turn off the TV. When Brian is transferred into my arms, I sense his body tension. I feel in my own body his efforts not to mold into my shoulder as I embrace him, instead orienting his gaze and whole body away from full-body contact with me. The rhythm of his breath is accelerated and shallow. Instinctually, I quiet my full-body actions, taking a deeper breath to complement his rhythm by decelerating my pace, taking one full breath within each of his four beats. This seems to help, as the rhythm of Brian's breathing begins to slow down. I quietly speak to him with a soft cadence, stating that I know he does not know me, but I am here to help, and we can take our time to get to know each other.

As his breath pace becomes more regulated, I introduce dancing together gently by experimenting with two actions: rocking with a subtle accented beat, and swaying with a slight flow side to side. I sense Brian responding to the sway. His body softens, and he places his head in the nook of my neck. We dance together like this for the next 10 minutes, and Brian falls asleep. This becomes the opening ritual for each subsequent DMT session with Brian.

Clinical Discussion

There are times when parents cannot be present for multiple hours during their child's hospitalization and the baby needs to be soothed by support staff. In Brian's case, Tortora engages him by focusing on how his biological and behavioral experiences are influencing his emotional expression. She observes Brian's emotional reactivity through his nonverbal cues before and during her engagement. First, she reduces his sensory input by shutting off the TV to remove the overstimulating sensations Brian was experiencing. Slowly, she layers in age-appropriate specific sensations to soothe him, providing an emotional connection rather than electronic stimulation. Using multisensory tools to support intrinsic and extrinsic regulatory domains, Tortora attunes to Brian's heightened arousal, evidenced by his increased breath rate, and behavioral attempts to self-soothe demonstrated by his gaze aversion and whole-body orienting away from the caregiver. Tortora adapts her behaviors to provide extrinsic support, adjusting her breathing rhythm to calm and center herself and create a body-to-body dialogue with Brian to organize their breath patterns. This shapes their engagement. By slowing the timing of her actions and eliminating other inputs, she patiently waits for Brian's embodied responses before adding another layer of novelty. Adding prosodic verbalizations, and then the swaying dance, culminates in Brian softening his body and resting his head into her shoulder. This provides a new soothing extrinsic, embodied experience that Brian can build on as he develops self-regulation, biologically and emotionally. This is an example of what Hofer discusses as the experiential nature of learning regulation.

This vignette also illustrates the impact of the parent's absence on the hospitalized child's emotional reactions. It is indeed common for parents – especially single parents and those of several children – to be in an emotional dilemma. When they are in the hospital caring for the sick child, they are not attending to their children at home, and vice versa. The next time Brian's mother is present, Tortora strikes a delicate balance between modeling how to soothe Brian and helping her feel competent in her understanding of her baby, despite her inability to be present all the time. Tortora does this by first emphasizing how much Brian knows Mom, evidenced in his immediate orientation to her, translating his whole-body movement toward her as a loving recognition of her presence. Tortora then enthusiastically describes Brian's ability to regulate his body while in her arms as *his* capacity to co-regulate. As Mom holds him, Tortora guides her through the nonverbal cues she has noted, teaching Mom how to pay attention to her own breathing and body tension in relationship to Brian. Sharing in this way supports Mom's self-confidence and creates a positive experience in the moment between them, contributing to their attachment relationship. These are elements of the Embodied Parenting program.

Embodied Parenting

The Embodied Parenting (EP) program supports the development of healthy attachment relationships, emphasizing the importance of the felt experiential exchange between the caregiver and their baby. It teaches caregivers how to observe the more subtle, nonverbal aspects of their communications (Tortora, 2015). EP draws conscious awareness to the nature and felt experience of the nonverbal exchange between the caregiver and the infant by attending to the immediate moment on somatic, kinesthetic, and sensorial levels. As exemplified in the vignette with Tortora and Brian, the experience in one's body acts as the organizing principle within the body–mind–emotional continuum. Both the caregiver's and the child's felt body experience is primary (Tortora, 2013). In EP, parents – and with medical illnesses, other caregivers engaged in the care of the baby – are guided to reflect on how experiences such as motion, posture, and multisensory sensation influence how their child processes his experience. This is revealed through his reactions, behaviors, and affect. These felt experiences are the primary ways that the baby feels and gets to know himself, from which a symbolic sense of self emerges on perceptual, cognitive, and emotional levels (Tortora, 2006). EP also guides caregivers to observe and reflect on what their own body sensations communicate to their baby and what these sensations reveal about their own conscious and unconscious present and past. From this level of self and other awareness, mutually attuned interactions called "dancing dialogues" are revealed (Tortora, 2006).

Understanding how the parent and infant's reactions and behaviors co-regulate each member of the dyad is a prominent focus in infant mental health, and an essential aspect of EP. Everyday life interactions between a parent and infant that include coordinated exchanges of mutual social-affective states create sequences of positive reciprocity. This mutual dance helps regulate dyadic members and build the parent's sense of competence in their parenting skill (Papoušek, 2011). Even before the infant can independently achieve state or emotion regulation, the child is biologically "prewired" with visual, vocal, and motor capacities that motivate the infant to engage with the parent. In return, the parent's biological nurturing instincts complement the infant's behaviors, compelling the parent to read and respond to the baby's nonverbal cues and emerging emotion and state behaviors, interpreting them as feeling states.

But extremely stressful situations can compromise this instinctual dynamic between parents and their babies, so EP provides a method to help parents observe and learn about their baby's temperamental style, emotion reactivity, and arousal, coping, and psychosocial regulatory skills within the context of how medical illness impacts their child's felt embodied experience and engagement and their own reactions. This occurs by understanding their child's and their own unique nonverbal cues. Through this focus on nonverbal communication, parents learn how to provide attuned nurturing responses contingent on their infant's needs. Dance and music activities that are culturally specific to the family are used to soothe and engage the young child, enhancing the dancing dialogue and supporting the developing attachment relationship. Indeed, recent research using a biobehavioral framework demonstrates that positive mother-and-child free play interactions create physiological and behavioral coordinations that contribute to the young child's socioemotional development (Hu et al., 2021).

The Neurobiological Basis of the Attachment Relationship and Its Link to Early Experience of Several Medical Illnesses

The innovative work of Hofer, quoted earlier in this chapter, has influenced the present interest in the neurobiological basis of the regulatory role created by the ongoing caregiver–infant relationship. With specific focus on the dynamics between the mother and infant, Hofer's term "hidden regulators" describes the effects the mother-infant social interaction has on the physiological, neurophysiological, behavioral, and emotional developmental processes of the infant (Hofer, 1995, p. 204). "Hidden" refers to the surprising regulatory consequences the mother's nurturing behavior has on the infant's multiple sensorimotor, thermal-metabolic, and nutrient-based mechanisms. These hidden regulators operate separately from psychological motivators, implying that something is happening on a deep physiological, body level that is separate from our conscious control. In the medical setting, we are particularly interested in those components of the parental nonverbal interactions that shape the development of the infant's behavior and biological and emotional systems, including the level and rate of touch, warmth, smell, physical proximity, and distancing, and how the infant senses the position and movement of their caregiver's limbs and body in space. Embodied Parenting provides a playful way to enhance these nonverbal behaviors, as they occur naturally when dancing with a baby. By attending to these actions of the caregiver with conscious awareness and observing the infant's responses to these qualities during hospitalization, we can support co-regulation and the developing bond.

Hu's research, mentioned previously, is significant for the intervention focus of this book because it is the first study to measure physiological and behavioral synchrony in real time during mother-and-child cooperative play. Particularly important to our focus is that this type of coordinated play has a co-regulatory effect: The mother's emotional and physical availability affects the baby's physiological system; and the child's behaviors and emotional display affect the mother's physiological arousal (Hu et al., 2021). Hu cites the work of Porges' polyvagal theory (Porges, 2011) to explain the regulatory role the sympathetic and parasympathetic branches of the autonomic nervous system play in affective processes and social functioning.

The polyvagal theory and polyvagal-informed therapy for trauma and attachment focus on the specific mechanisms that our nervous system uses to detect risk or safety as they affect our physiological and behavioral states. Safety in polyvagal theory is demarcated by body responses rather than cognitive appraisal; "the 'wisdom' resides in our body and in the structures of our nervous system that function outside the realm of awareness" (Porges, 2017, p. 43). Porges created the term "neuroception" to describe the process in which the nervous system evaluates risk involving cues for danger, safety, or life threat, operating out of our conscious awareness (Porges, 2004, 2011). Neuroception triggers physiological states felt through interoception that create emotional responses of trust or danger. A sense of danger activates the defensive strategies of mobilization, related to fighting or fleeing, or immobilization, which involves states of hiding or feigning death.

Focusing on the parasympathetic vague system, Porges states that from birth "humans are on a quest to calm neural defense systems by detecting features of safety" (Porges & Daniel, 2017, p. 114). He cites the engagement of the vagus nerve, known as vagal tone, as the safety response detector. Vagal nerve engagement or withdrawal is measured by the amplitude of respiratory sinus arrhythmia (RSA), the metric used to indicate the rhythmic heart rate which naturally increases and decreases in synchrony with breathing. When an individual is in a safe co-regulated state with another person, vagal tone is active, acting as a vagal brake with increases in heart rate variability (HRV) by increasing intervals between heartbeats through longer exhalations. Increased HRV is linked to physical and mental adaptability, supporting healthy adaptive social behavior; decreased HRV represents a vulnerability to stress. When distressed, the fight-or-flight autonomic stress response is activated, marked by vagal withdrawal, decreasing RSA/HRV and reducing parasympathetic activity and social behavior.

Vagal activity measured through HRV was used in Suga's recent research to understand how the enhancement of vagal tone activity might support growth and socioemotional development (Suga et al., 2019). They found that vagal activity in babies can be enhanced by influencing a mother's HRV through slow-paced, diaphragmatic breathing, and that vocal synchrony between mothers and their 3-month-old infants during face-to-face engagement coordinated their heart rhythms. As is demonstrated throughout this book, Embodied Parenting intervention activities support the caregiver to use their breath, voice, and whole body to create synchronized and coordinated playful interactions to soothe and engage their babies.

The polyvagal theory emphasizes that the primary caregiver's ability to create a co-regulating state – necessary for the development of a trusting, safe, secure attachment relationship – exists by accurately detecting signals of comfort or distress, which are often transmitted though postures, gestures, and other nonverbal cues. Facial expressivity and vocal tone are specifically referenced as key ways safety is detected on a neurobiological level. Porges (2017, p. xv) states that social behavior is "defined by a face-heart connection in which the neural regulation of the striated muscles of our face and head are neurophysiologically linked to the neural regulation of our heart." During social engagements, this face/heart connection is what enables us to truly soothe a loved one, calming their physiological state. Porges' work highlights the reciprocal relationship between the neurophysiological interpretations of safety and the psychosocial felt experience of the individual. This is very relevant to the context of the infant's and parents' experience when the baby is hospitalized with a severe medical illness, as their attachment system is triggered by the stressful, unfamiliar situation, and reading and responding to the subtle meaning of the caregivers' and the child's nonverbal cues can be compromised.

Conclusion

As stated by Clancy and her colleagues, in the context of the psychosocial development of children with congenital heart disease (CHD), there is a lack of understanding of the short- and long-term emotion and behavioral regulation of young children with medical illness. It is essential for the well-being of children with chronic and critical illness that we contemplate how they each develop self-regulatory capacities, cope with stress, and acquire social skills. "Gaining an understanding of early psychosocial development is important to sensitize clinicians to the young child's distress and to inform clinical care from diagnosis onwards" (Clancy et al., 2019, p. 3).

This chapter provides an overview of key theories and research to advance our understanding of the complex factors that influence the young child's embodied experience as it affects their psychosocial development and attachment relationships. The research provided explains how parents and significant caregivers influence the infant and young child's physiological, psychological, and behavioral development of self-regulation. Hidden regulators in the parent–infant interaction play a crucial role in shaping development within the context of the relationship. In polyvagal theory, feeling safe is instrumental to regulation and healing, and a lack of safety can result in mental and physical illness on a biobehavioral level. Porges' approach emphasizes the importance of the embodied experience of social relationships and provides a neurophysiological basis for the foundational principles of attachment theory. These principles support the embodied, felt experiences at the core of pediatric medical DMT intervention. EP offers a method for parents and medical practitioners to observe the nonverbal cues of young children to support self-regulation, engagement, and coping during their illness.

The caregiver's ability to accurately respond to the baby's cues with specific behaviors – such as holding the crying baby to achieve a calm state and providing a soothing, regulated presence that encourages the baby's explorations – can be instrumental in creating an embodied sense of safety that supports the attachment–exploration continuum for a medically ill baby. One immediate application of this work is to encourage parents to take the role of providing emotional support solely through their embodied interactions with the baby. Soothing their child during and after procedures, rather than holding their child during the procedures, preserves their protective role. Hearing a parent's loving voice, gazing at a parent's warm facial expressions during a procedure, and being held and rocked by the parent afterward maintain the parent's role as a secure, soothing base on a deeply psychological and physiological level. When parents or other significant caregivers in the child's life can't be present, specially designated medical team member(s) can take on this sensitive regulating role during difficult procedures and also facilitate and maintain an embodied sense of safety for the infant.

References

Barlow, J., Herath, NINS., Bartram, T., Bennett, C., & Wei, Y. (2018). The neonateal behavioral assessment scale (NBAS) and the newborn behavioral observations (NBO) system for supporting caregivers and improving outcomes in caregivers and their infants (Review). *Cochrane Database of Systematic Reviews* (3), Article CD011754. https://doi org/10.1002/14651858.CD011754.pub2. (John Wiley & Sons, Ltd.)

Bates, J., & Pettit, A. (2015). Temperament, parenting, and social development. In J. Grusec & P. Hastings (Eds.), *Handbook of socialization: Theory and research* (pp. 372–397). The Guilford Press.

Bates, J., Schermerhorn, A., & Petersen, I. (2012). Temperament and parenting in developmental perspective. In M. Zentner & R. Shiner (Eds.), *Handbook of temperament* (pp. 425–441). Guildford Press.

Bowlby, J. (1969). *Attachment and loss: Volume 1. Attachment*. Basic Books.

Braungart-Rieker, J., Hill-Soderlund, A., & Karrass, J. (2010). Fear and anger reactivity trajectories from 4 to 16 months: The roles of temperament, regulation, and maternal sensitivity. *Developmental Psychology, 46*(4), 791–804. https://doi.org/doi.org/10.1037/a0019673

Calkins, S., & Hill, A. (2006). Caregiver influences on emerging emotion regulation: Biological and environmental transactions in early development. In J. Gross (Ed.), *Handbook of emotion regulation: First Edition* (1st ed.). Guilford Publications.

Carey, W., & Me Devitt, S. (1978). Revision of the infant temperament questionnaire. *Pediatrics, 61*, 735–739.

Cassidy, J., Woodhouse, S. S., Cooper, G., Hoffman, K., Powell, B., & Rodenberg, M. (2005). Examination of the precursors of infant attachment security: Implications for early intervention and intervention research. In Y. Z. L. J. Berlin, L. Amaya-Jackson, &

M. T. Greenberg (Eds.), *Enhancing early attachments: Theory, research, intervention, and policy* (pp. 34–60). Guilford.

Chen, X., & Schmidt, L. (2015). Temperament and personality. In M. Lamb & R. Lerner (Eds.), *Social, emotional, and personality development. Volume 3 of the Handbook of child psychology and developmental science* (Vol. 7, pp. xx–xx). Wiley.

Chess, S., & Thomas, A. (1997). Temperamental individuality from childhood to adolescence. *Journal of American Academy of Child Psychiatry*, *16*(2), 218–226.

Clancy, T., Jordan, B., de Weerth, C., & Muscara, F. (2019, 2019/09/10). Early emotional, behavioural and social development of infants and young children with congenital heart disease: A systematic review. *Journal of Clinical Psychology in Medical Settings*. https://doi.org/10.1007/s10880-019-09651-1

DeGangi, G., Breinbauer, C., Doussard Roosevelt, J., Porges, S., & Greenspan, S. (2000). Prediction of childhood problems at three years in children experiencing disorders of regulation during infancy. *Journal of Infant Mental Health*, *21*(3), 156–175. https://doi.org/10.1002/1097-0355(200007)21

Gross, J. (2013a). Emotion regulation: Conceptual and empirical foundations. In J. Gross (Ed.), *Handbook of emotion regulation* (2nd ed., pp. 3–20). Guildford Press.

Gross, J. (2013b). Emotion regulation: Taking stock and moving forward. *Emotion*, *13*(3), 359–265.

Hofer, M. (1995). Hidden regulators: Implications for a new understanding of attachment, separation, and loss. In S. Goldberg, R. Muir, & J. Kerr (Eds.), *Attachment theory: Social, developmental, and clinical perspectives* (pp. 203–230). The Analytic Press.

Hu, Y., McElwain, N., & Berry, D. (2021). Mother – child mutually responsive orientation and real-time physiological coordination. *Developmental Psychobiology*, *63*(7), e22200. https://doi.org/https://doi.org/10.1002/dev.22200

Papoušek, M. (2011). Resilience, strengths, and regulatory capacities: Hidden resources in developmental disorders of infant mental health. *Infant Mental Health Journal*, *32*(1), 29–46.

Park, S. Y., Belsky, J., Putnam, S., & Crnic, K. (1997, Mar). Infant emotionality, parenting, and 3-year inhibition: Exploring stability and lawful discontinuity in a male sample. *Developmental Psychology*, *33*(2), 218–227. https://doi.org/10.1037//0012-1649.33.2.218

Pauli-Pott, U., Mertesacker, B., & Beckmann, D. (2004, Winter). Predicting the development of infant emotionality from maternal characteristics. *Development and Psychopathology*, *16*(1), 19–42. https://doi.org/10.1017/S0954579404044396

Porges, S. W. (2004). Neuroception: A subconcious system for detecting threats and safety. *Zero to Three*, *24*(5), 19–24.

Porges, S. W. (2011). *The polyvagal theory: Neurophysiological foundations of emotions, attachment, communication and self-regulation*. W. W. Norton & Co., Inc.

Porges, S. W. (2017). *The pocket guide to the polyvagal theory: The transformative power of feeling safe*. W. W. Norton Press & Company.

Porges, S. W., & Daniel, S. (2017). Play and dynamics of treating pediatric medical trauma. In S. Daniel & C. Trevarthen (Eds.), *Rhythms of relating in children's therapies: Connecting creatively with vunerable children* (pp. 113–124). Jessica Kingsley Publishers.

Rothbart, M. K. (1981). Measurement of temperament in infancy. *Child Development*, *52*, 569–578. https://doi.org/10.2307/1129176.

Rothbart, M. K. (2011). *Becoming who we are*. Guilford.

Rothbart, M. K., Sheese, B. E., Rueda, M. R., & Posner, M. I. (2011). Developing mechanisms of self-regulation in early life. *Emotion Review: Journal of the International Society for Research on Emotion*, *3*(2), 207–213. https://doi.org/10.1177/1754073910387943

Sameroff, A. J., & MacKenzie, M. J. (2003). Capturing transactional models of development: The limits of the possible. *Development & Psychopathology*, *15*, 613–640.

Shiner, R., Buss, K., McClowry, S., Putnam, S., Saudino, K., & Zentner, M. (2012). What is temperament now? *Child Development Perspectives*, *6*, 436–444. https://doi.org/10.1111/j.1750-8606.2012.00254.x.

Suga, A., Uraguchi, M., Tange, A., Ishikawa, H., & Ohira, H. (2019, 2019/12/27). Cardiac interaction between mother and infant: Enhancement of heart rate variability. *Scientific Reports*, *9*(1), 20019. https://doi.org/10.1038/s41598-019-56204-5

Tortora, S. (2006). *The dancing dialogue: Using the communicative power of movement with young children*. Paul H. Brookes Publishing Company.

Tortora, S. (2013). The essential role of the body in the parent-infant relationship: Nonverbal analysis of attachment. In J. F. Bettmann (Ed.), *Attachment-based clinical social work with children and adolescents* (pp. 141–164). Springer.

Tortora, S. (2015). The importance of being seen – Winnicott, dance movement psychotherapy and the embodied experience. In M. Spelman & F. Thomson-Salo (Eds.), *The Winnicott tradition: Lines of development – evolution of theory and practice over the decades*. Karnac.

Wiefferink, C. H., Rieffe, C., Ketelaar, L., & Frijns, J. H. (2012, Jun). Predicting social functioning in children with a cochlear implant and in normal-hearing children: The role of emotion regulation. *International Journal of Pediatric Otorhinolaryngology*, *76*(6), 883–889. https://doi.org/10.1016/j.ijporl.2012.02.065

Wolff, P. (1987). *The development of behavioral states and the expression of emotions in early infancy*. The University of Chicago Press.

Woodhouse, S., Scott, J., Hepworth, A., & Cassidy, J. (2019). Secure base provision: A new approach to examining links between maternal caregiving and infant attachment. *Child Development*, 1–17. https://doi.org/10.1111/cdev.13224

Zeanah, C. (2019). *Handbook of infant mental health* (C. Zeanah, Ed., 4th ed.). The Guildford Press.

Chapter 5

Babies Remember Pain

Nathan is 21 months old at the time of referral to our Infant Mental Health Clinic because of food refusal. When he was born, he was diagnosed with a severe genetic skin disease, Netherton syndrome, an autosomal-recessive disease characterized by massive ichthyosis, recurrent skin infections, continuous itching, scars, thin hair, various degrees of failure to thrive, and intellectual disability. Nathan's delivery was difficult and traumatic. He spent his first three months of life in the neonatal intensive care unit in total isolation due to fear of life-threatening infection. Nobody was allowed to touch him because any infection was potentially deadly.

Nathan's appearance is painful to look at: His skin looks similar to that of a person with third-degree burns; his mouth opening is so small that he can be fed only through gastrostomy. He can hardly cry and never smiles. Nathan has a stern look in his eyes and sits motionless. Although there is no specific medical reason for the absence of crawling, Nathan seems as if he is imprisoned in his own body. He scratches himself in complete silence, absorbed in his painful body.

As Nathan is withdrawn within his endless pain, his parents are also withdrawn into their own grief over the healthy baby who was not born. The tension between the parents is observable. Their relationship had been stressed before Nathan's birth, and his illness has created more tension. The father has withdrawn from his child and the mother has withdrawn from her husband. Mother becomes focused on the child only; she stops working and restricts her life.

Both parents are present during our meetings, as part of the treatment focus includes improving the parents' dynamics, but the tension is palpable. Touching on the matter of their infant's illness with words is as painful as concretely touching the infant. Nathan's stillness reminds us of Fraiberg's (1982) notion of freezing, one of the pathological defenses she observed in very frightened infants. Nathan's symptoms of depression include a severe developmental arrest, food refusal, no psychomotor exploration, lack of vitality, and withdrawal from interpersonal interactions. Nathan's mother has concealed her own depression, which started with her son's birth.

DOI: 10.4324/9781003134800-6

Clinical Discussion

The specific family constellation in Nathan's case requires the medical team to be very careful in how they approach these complex issues. The psychotherapeutic treatment must be organized to support the family and child. The child's rare congenital syndrome adds a significant stress to the parents' already challenged relationship, preventing them from supporting each other. The first thing Keren does is to establish the link between the child's experience of physical pain and his poor development. Initially, Mother is convinced that the child is mainly mentally compromised and does not appreciate the impact of the pain his skin causes him. Nathan's external appearance resembles that of a third-degree burn patient, and he has extreme pain when his skin peels off. Looking at him and touching him is difficult, causing the parents to feel repulsed by him. Being able to talk about these profoundly negative feelings is the main therapeutic task, as Mom does not feel that she has permission to feel this way. She tries to hide these feelings and thoughts. She feels like a monster mom of a monster baby. Keren can identify with these feelings of repulsion, because it is so difficult to look at Nathan as his skin oozes viscous liquid.

To counteract these reactions and to help Nathan feel an embodied sense of engagement, Keren sits on the floor, at his level, and leans toward him. She finds it easier to focus on his face, especially his eyes, than to look at his whole body. Nathan can hardly smile because his skin is so tight. Keren addresses the pain: "It must be painful for you every day, especially when you have to take so many baths, and then get dressed. Mom can feel your pain as well, but sometimes she doesn't know what to do." Mom is very surprised to hear Keren talking about the pain, because she had not thought to directly approach this aspect of her son's condition. It helps her to see that Keren is not as afraid of the situation and that she can take in the whole dynamic, including Mom's ambivalence toward Nathan.

Not addressing the pain directly complicates the caregiving relationship and the child's whole development. Nathan's clinical presentation of his distress had remained undiagnosed for months. The medical staff had not been aware of the extremely detrimental impact chronic, severe pain and the damaged skin envelope had on Nathan's development. The impact of the genetic disease on the early parent–infant relationship had also not been assessed. Improvement in the infant's condition starts with the process of making the link between the child's physical pain and his developmental arrest, at first with his pediatrician and his parents, and then with him in the room. Talking about the impact of pain in a direct and simple manner by acknowledging that Nathan feels bad in his body, and that this makes him sad and angry, is helpful for the parents and child. Nathan explores more, his eyes become brighter, and he eats better after this treatment.

Introduction

There was a time in recent history when it was thought that babies could not remember pain or any preverbal experiences due to a lack of cognitive and language skills. It was only in 1993 that medical doctors started to point out how very young children do recall pain (Gauvain-Piquard & Meignier, 1993). Withdrawal and muteness were the reactions they observed and understood as an autistic-like defense, as illustrated in the opening vignette of this chapter. Today, the standard approach is to prescribe analgesics medication, like we do for older children. Premature babies' sensory experience in the neonatal intensive care unit (NICU) – including exposure to bright lights, high sound levels, and frequent noxious interventions – may exert deleterious effects on the immature brain and alter its subsequent development (Als et al., 2004). The importance of syncing environment and the brain's expectation during "critical" periods of brain development has long been demonstrated in animal models of development (Wiesel & Hubel, 1965). In an effort to decrease the discrepancy between the immature human brain's expectation and the actual experience in a typical NICU, a comprehensive approach was developed, the Newborn Individualized Developmental Care and Assessment Program (NIDCAP), and found to be effective in improving neurodevelopmental outcomes for premature babies (Buehler et al., 1995).

Additional studies in the domain of trauma and PTSD in the pediatric population have demonstrated that traumatic experiences, especially early childhood ones, are stored in lower parts of the brain and can be triggered by multisensory stimulations many years later (Taddio et al., 2002; Puchalski & Hummel, 2002; van der Kolk, 2015; Perry & Pollard, 1998).

Chronic pain, medically unexplained symptoms, and somatization syndromes in adults have indeed been associated with early traumas, including early medical conditions that compromised the parent–infant relationship (Coates, 2016). In particular, chronic pain linked with medical procedures may challenge and compromise the infant's developing neuroceptive capacity for self-regulation (Porges, 2007).

Besides the impact of the pain experience, anticipatory distress with recurrent painful procedures is now well recognized among children of all ages. Four types of factors have been related to anticipatory distress (Racine et al., 2016): predisposing (e.g. genetics and temperament), precipitating (e.g. negative pain experiences), perpetuating (e.g. parent behavior, parent situational and anticipatory anxiety that is increased by parent's previous pain experience, child behavior, and child maladaptive cognitions such as perceived loss of control and threat appraisal), and present (e.g. health care and professional behavior, rather than hospitalization by itself). For instance, young age and a difficult, fearful temperament are factors that increase the risk of a child's anticipatory distress. In this chapter, we elucidate how the bulk of recent knowledge specifically relates to the baby's experience of illness-related pain, with a focus on what needs to be assessed and treated.

Infants Do Remember Pain and Context

In an article entitled "The Birth of Consciousness" (Lagercrantz, 2009), newborns are depicted as being able to differentiate between self- and non–self–touch and to process sensory impressions at a cortical level. The article posits that newborns remember rhythmic sounds and vowels they were exposed to during fetal life. When presented with these sounds after birth, newborns demonstrate a spontaneous resting activity in their cortex, indicating they are reacting and remembering sounds they were familiar with in utero.

Pain is both an affective and sensory experience, and the infant will remember both via his implicit memory network (Taddio et al., 2002). On the sensory level, signs of pain in a critically ill infant may be subtle, such as an imperceptible movement or a sudden gaze change. Thus, the infant's pain experience has long been underestimated, the general thought being that the infant is too young to feel pain. But in recent years, monitoring and neuroimaging techniques – such as cerebral near-infrared spectroscopy as a measure of nociceptive evoked activity in very ill infants – have become more common in pain research (Ranger et al., 2011). With repeated painful experiences, permanent structural and function changes occur in the brain and spinal cord, and adverse neurodevelopmental outcomes are described. Infants remember pain and, consequently, react differently to subsequent painful experiences. They may withdraw or become irritable or extremely anxious and clingy. In light of this emerging evidence, pediatricians, especially neonatologists and surgeons, have become increasingly aware of the reality of neonatal pain (Puchalski & Hummel, 2002).

From a developmental perspective, the affective component of the pain experience and memory for the infant linked with the extent to which he felt physical and emotional closeness with a parent during times of pain. Indeed, the sociocommunication model of infant pain (Craig & Pillai Riddell, 2003) suggests that the infant-pain paradigm cannot be fully understood outside of the caregiving context, given that the infant and caregiver are separately influenced by the larger ecological system of family, culture, and community. The model describes four stages: the painful event that triggers the experience of infant pain, the infant's expression of pain, the sensitive caregiver assessing the nonverbal expression of pain, and the caregiver taking soothing action. Inherent in this model is the complexity of some clinical situations where the caregiver's past pain-related and non–pain-related interactions impact the quality of the caregiver's reactions to the infant's pain.

We can use the concept of "schema of being" (Stern, 1994, p. 9), the inner representation of an interpersonal repeated experience at cognitive and affective levels, to conceptualize how the infant may develop an inner representation of the pain experience as a "schema of being with caregiver when I am in pain." Stern explores how an infant might represent object-related, interpersonal experience, and proposes that these moments are represented in at least six separate, parallel, basic schematic formats: sensorimotor, perceptions, concepts, scripts, temporal feeling shapes, and proto-narrative envelopes. The temporal feeling shape is proposed as a format for representing affects, and the proto-narrative envelope is proposed as a format for representing the global experience in a narrative, like form. Taken together, these six formats comprise a network of schemas that we call the "schema of being with."

A recent study (Noel et al., 2017) examined parent–child reminiscence of a recent painful surgery in the pain-memory development of young children. The findings revealed that a more elaborate parental reminiscing style, together with a greater use of emotional words, predicted more accurate and positive pain memories; greater parental use of pain-related words predicted more negative memories. Mothers and fathers differed in how they reminisced, but no gender or parent-role differences were linked to the child's pain-memory biases. In another very recent study (Fischer et al., 2019), a parent trait anxiety profile (meaning anxious personality) predicted more negatively biased memories for pain-related fear; a parent state anxiety level profile (meaning anxiety that is provoked by the child's illness) and child preoperative anxiety level did not.

Even when pain has been experienced as an acute and isolated experience, such as after a surgery, its impact does not necessarily end when the pain does: Pain memories are vulnerable to distortion. Children's catastrophic thinking about pain – to magnify it, for example – increases its threatening aspect, which leads to more distressing pain memories. Also, parents' catastrophic thinking – such as rumination and helplessness – impacts the child's pain experience negatively. This leads parents to develop more distressing memories about their child's pain. Parent and child catastrophizing have been associated with persistent post-surgical pain (Noel et al., 2017).

This new understanding of the extent to which pain continues after the procedure ends (Noel et al., 2012) has even more clinical significance in situations of chronic severe medical illness, when the infant accumulates pain-related memories and experiences during treatment. Fifty-five children, ages 3–18, were tested for their memories of lumbar punctures; results showed that children of all ages displayed considerable accuracy in recalling event details, a capacity that increased with age (Chen et al., 2000). Higher distress predicted greater exaggerations in negative memory one week later, which predicted higher distress at a subsequent lumbar puncture.

Pain as a Potential Toxic Stressor for the Infant's Developing Brain

In contrast with routine immunizations, repeated exposure to non-normative painful procedures, such as those inherent in serious illness, engenders stress, which will be tolerable or toxic depending on the buffering presence of a caregiver to help the infant cope and reduce the physiological stress response. Toxic stress has been defined as an experience that produces frequent, strong, and/or prolonged activation of the body stress response system in the absence of a supportive infant-caregiver relationship (Kroupina & Elison, 2019). It affects metabolic systems, brain circuitry, and the child's cognitive and socioemotional development (Shonkoff & Garner, 2012). The plasticity of the developing brain implies that toxic stress has dramatic neurological effects in the first three years of life, with the detrimental effects of early toxic stress involving three regions of the brain: the amygdala, hippocampus, and the prefrontal cortex (Boyce & Ellis, 2005). Although we do not yet have the ability to predict the impact of severe pain-related stress on individual infants, our role is to find those infants who lack a supportive relationship with their caregiver and are at high risk for experiencing toxic stress.

Assessing the Infant's Pain Expressions

Knowing that infants remember pain and experience it as a significant stressor tasks the medical team with assessing the infant's pain expressions, which is difficult because infants are obviously unable to verbalize their pain. Infants are totally dependent on adults, so caregivers play a crucial role in determining the extent of the infant's pain in order to take appropriate action to manage it (Pillai Riddell & Racine, 2009). Idiosyncratic variables that impact empathy and helping someone in pain include cognitive processes, like intentionality, pain experiences, and interpersonal judgment (Goubert et al., 2005). In the case of infants in pain, it is especially important to consider what the assessor, parents, physicians, and nurses bring into the judgment context.

Different caregivers bring different beliefs and experiences to this context, as shown in three different studies (Pillai Riddell et al., 2004; Pillai Riddell & Craig, 2007; Pillai Riddell et al., 2008). Despite every group being shown the same infants with the same level of pain expression, significant differences were observed among caregiver groups: Parents attributed the highest pain level to the infants, pediatricians the lowest, and nurses in the middle, regardless of the infant's age (from 2–18 months). It is important to note that higher pain judgments may not translate to better management of the infant's pain. For example, pediatricians had significantly more optimal beliefs regarding the appropriateness of pain medication for babies than parents. To make things even more complicated, the infant's caregivers may magnify or moderate the child's pain-related distress (Cramer-Berness, 2007), so it is of paramount importance to understand the reciprocal relationship between infant and parent behaviors when assessing infant pain. For instance, a measure that evaluates soothing sensitive parental behaviors in the pain context should be defined by an infant's positive reaction, meaning lower distress reactivity, rather than judging parental soothing behaviors as sensitive. Some infants in pain are soothed by rocking, others are not, even though rocking may be generally considered a sensitive behavior.

Pain, Body Trauma, and Later-Life Symptoms in Adulthood

Children who have undergone painful or traumatic early medical experiences are more vulnerable to pain conditions as adults, diagnosed as chronic pain, medically unexplained symptoms (MUS), and somatization spectrum disorders (SSD) (Anderson, 2017). The research and literature in trauma treatment is based on the understanding that trauma is stored in the body, resulting in physiological and psychological changes, which respond to treatment methods that enable the reintegration of the body, mind, and emotions, including therapies that incorporate body- and movement-oriented activities (van der Kolk, 2015). Using the body to retrieve memories, including autobiographical ones, has shown that memories can be embodied through body postures (Dijkstra et al., 2007). This research demonstrates that when subjects are prompted during retrieval of a past event to take on the specific posture of that event, they display better free recall and faster response times.

Taking this embodied memory recall research a step further, a study on metaphorical mental representation reveals that subjects remember more positive memories when moving their arms upward and more negative memories when moving them downward (Casasanto & Dijkstra, 2010). This has led researchers to conclude that analogous to action simulation processes, apparatuses for emotional simulation also exist (Jung & Sparenberg, 2012). These studies have implications for the use of movement – and of specific dynamics in actions – as potentially powerful tools in the treatment of trauma.

Clinical Implications

Today, it is common practice to give newborns and infants anesthesia before painful procedures. A study on children undergoing cancer procedures under pharmacological sedation (Dufresne et al., 2010) has shown that sedation is indeed effective in lowering the child's levels of fear and pain during procedures, but it does not alleviate stress before the next procedure. In the study sample, children anticipating high levels of pain and fear experienced higher levels of pain. Furthermore, in older children, it was found that sedation impacts explicit memory but not implicit memory (Pringle et al., 2003), which is nonverbal and mostly unconscious. Implicit memory is already present in the last trimester of pregnancy and is predominant in infancy, in contrast with explicit memory, which emerges by the age of 18 months and develops with the acquisition of language. These findings are very significant, revealing that sedation does not prevent the infant from developing aversive implicit memories, especially when she is severely medically compromised and experiences pain over a long time period. This is also the reason why body-, dance-, and movement-oriented interventions are so relevant in addressing these felt memories.

Conclusion

All experiences change the brain, but not all experiences affect the brain equally. Because the brain is developing and organizing at such an explosive rate in the first years of life, experiences during this period have more potential to influence the brain in positive and negative ways. Traumatic events disrupt homeostasis in multiple areas of the brain that are recruited to respond to the threat. Use-dependent internalization of elements of the traumatic experience can result in the persistence of fear-related neurophysiologic patterns affecting emotional, behavioral, cognitive, and social functioning. Chronic or repeated experience with pain may become a toxic stress for the infant, both physiologically and psychologically, putting him at risk for later development of mental and physical disorders. The current knowledge about existing implicit memory, even before birth, no longer allows us to think that babies do not remember pain and therefore are not at risk.

Children in the first three years of life are more vulnerable to toxic stress, but they are also more sensitive to the positive impact of early interventions. In light of what we mentioned previously, the major tenet of pain-related intervention is to try to keep the pain experience tolerable by fostering a supportive caregiver-infant relationship. Whatever method is used to work on the parent–infant relationship, assessment of the infant's characteristics and the caregivers' own past history of traumas and pain-related experiences are necessary for planning the intervention.

References

Als, H., Duffy, F. H., McAnultry, G., Rivkin, M., Vajapeyam, S., Mulkern, R., et al. (2004). Early experience alters brain function and structure. *Pediatrics* (113), 846–857.

Anderson, F. (2017). It was not safe to feel angry: Disruptive early attachment and the development of chronic pain in later life. *ATTACHMENT: New Directions in Psychotherapy and Relational Psychoanalysis, 11*, 223–241.

Boyce, W., & Ellis, B. (2005). Biological sensitivity to context: I. An evolutionary – developmental theory of the origins and functions of stress reactivity. *Development and Psychopathology*, *17*, 271–301.

Buehler, D., Als, H., Duffy, F., McAnulty, G., & Liederman, J. (1995). Effectiveness of individualized developmental care for low-risk preterm infants: Behavioral and electrophysiological evidence. *Pediatrics*, *96*, 923–932.

Casasanto, D., & Dijkstra, K. (2010). Motor action and emotional memory. *Cognition*, *115*(1), 179–185.

Chen, E., Zeltzer, L., Craske, M., & Katz, E. (2000). Children's memories for painful cancer treatment procedures: Implications for distress. *Child Development*, *71*, 933–947.

Coates, S. (2016). Can babies remember trauma? Symbolic forms of representation in traumatized infants. *Journal of American Psychoanalytical Association*, *64*, 751–776.

Craig, K., & Pillai Riddell, R. (2003). Social influences, culture and ethnicity. In G. Finley & P. McGrath (Eds.), *Pediatric pain: Biological and social context*. IASP Press.

Cramer-Berness, L. (2007). Development of the distraction for infant immunizations: The progress and challenges. *Children's Health Care*, *36*, 203–217.

Dijkstra, K., Kaschak, M., & Zwaan, R. (2007). Body posture facilitates retrieval of autobiographical memories. *Cognition*, *102*(1), 139–149.

Dufresne, A., Dugas, M., Samson, Y., Barré, P., Turcot, L., & Marc, I. (2010). Do children undergoing cancer procedures under pharmacological sedation still report pain and anxiety? A preliminary study. *Pain Medicine*, *11*, 215–223.

Fischer, S., Vinall, J., Pavlova, M., Graham, S., Jordan, A., Chorney, J., Rasic, N., Brookes, J., Hoy, M., Yunker, W., & Noel, M. (2019). Role of anxiety in young children's pain memory development after surgery. *Pain*, *160*, 965–972.

Fraiberg, S. (1982). Pathological defences in infancy. *Psychoanalytical Quaterly*, *4*, 612–635.

Gauvain-Piquard, A., & Meignier, M. (1993). *La douleur de l'enfant {The Child's Pain}*. Calmann-Levy.

Goubert, L., Craig, K., Vervoort, T., Morley, S., Sullivan, M., Williams, D. C., Cano, A., & Crombez, G. (2005). Facing others in pain: The effects of empathy. *Pain*, *118*, 285–288.

Jung, C., & Sparenberg, P. (2012). Cognitive perspectives on embodiment. In S. Koch, T. Fuchs, M. Summa, & C. Muller (Eds.), *Body memory, metaphor and movement* (pp. 141–154). John Bejamins Publishing Company.

Kroupina, M., & Elison, K. (2019, July). The pediatric birth to three clinic and early childhood mental health program, meeting the needs of complex pediatric patients. *Zero to Three*, 31–34.

Lagercrantz, H. (2009). The birth of consciousness. *Early Human Development*, *85*, S57–58.

Noel, M., Chambers, C., Petter, M., McGrath, P., Klein, R., & Stewart, S. (2012). Pain is not over when the needle ends: A review and preliminary model of acute pain memory development in childhood. *Pain Management*, *2*, 487–497.

Noel, M., Rabbitts, J., Fales, J., Chorney, J., & Palermo, T. (2017). The influence of pain memories on children's and adolescents' post-surgical pain experience: A longitudinal dyadic analysis. *Health Psychology*, *36*, 987–995.

Perry, B., & Pollard, R. (1998). Homeostasis, stress, trauma, and adaptation. A neurodevelopmental view of childhood trauma. *Child & Adolescent Psychiatry Clinics of North America*, *7*, 33–51.

Pillai Riddell, R., Badali, M., & Craig, K. (2004). Parental judgments of infant pain: Importance of perceived cognitive abilities, behavioural cues and contextual cues. *Pain Research and Management*, *9*, 73–80.

Pillai Riddell, R., & Craig, K. (2007). Judgments of infant pain: The impact of caregiver identity and infant age. *Journal of Pediatric Psychology*, *32*, 501–511.

Pillai Riddell, R., Horton, R., Hillgrove, J., & Craig, K. (2008). Caregiver beliefs underlying infant pain judgments: Contrasts of parents, nurses and pediatricians. *Pain Research and Management*, *13*, 489–496.

Pillai Riddell, R., & Racine, N. (2009). Assessing pain in infancy: The caregiver context. *Pain Research and Management*, *14*, 27–32.

Porges, S. (2007). The polyvagal perspective. *Biological Psychology*, *4*, 116–143.

Pringle, B., Dahlquist, L., & Eskenazi, A. (2003). Memory in pediatric patients undergoing conscious sedation for aversive medical procedures. *Health Psychology*, *22*, 263–269.

Puchalski, M., & Hummel, P. (2002). The reality of neonatal pain. *Advances in Neonatal Care*, *2*, 233–244.

Racine, N., Pillai Riddell, R., Khan, M., Calic, M., Taddio, A., & Tablon, P. (2016). Systematic review: Predisposing, precipitating, perpetuating, and present factors predicting anticipatory distress to painful medical procedures in children. *Journal of Pediatric Psychology*, *42*, 159–181.

Ranger, M., Johnston, C., Limperopoulos, C., Rennick, J., & du Plessis, A. (2011). Cerebral near-infrared spectroscopy as a measure of nociceptive evoked activity in critically ill infants. *Pain Research and Management*, *16*, 331–336.

Shonkoff, J., & Garner, A. (2012). The lifelong effects of early childhood adversity and toxic stress. *Pediatrics*, *129*, 232–246.

Stern, D. (1994). One way to build a clinically relevant baby. *Infant Mental Health Journal*, *15*, 9–25.

Taddio, A., Shah, V., Gilbert-MacLeod, C., & Katz, J. (2002). Conditioning and hyperalgesia in newborns exposed to repeated heel lances. *Journal of American Medical Association*, *288*, 857–861.

van der Kolk, B. (2015). *The body keeps the score: Brain, mind and body in the healing of trauma*. Penguin Books.

Wiesel, T., & Hubel, D. (1965). Comparison of the effects of unilateral and bilateral eye closure on cortical unit responses in kittens. *Journal of Neurophysiology*, *28*, 1029–1040.

Chapter 6

The Hospital and Severe Illness-Linked Experiences

Their Impact on the Infant's Socioemotional Development

Charlie, a 3-year-old boy with chronic renal failure, is assigned to me (Keren) for a psychiatric consultation because he refused oral feeding. He has been fed through a percutaneous endoscopic gastrostomy (PEG) since he was 9 months old. Because of Charlie's refusal of oral intake, he did not reach the minimal weight required for the kidney transplant he needs. His kidney failure is part of a syndrome that includes congenital blindness, and he has been on dialysis for a year.

In my first encounter with Charlie, I am struck by the intensity of the anxiety he displays when I get closer to him, as if he anticipates another painful procedure. He screams, feeling my presence without seeing me.

He calms down slightly when I explain to him that I am a "doctor of feelings" and that I will not touch him. His parents are surprised by his reaction to my words, realizing for the first time how intense their child's anticipatory anxiety is due to repeated experiences with painful procedures compounded by his blindness.

Clinical Discussion

Anticipatory anxiety is very common, yet we must wonder why the option of talking to Charlie about the link between his anxiety, the medical procedures he has experienced, and in this case, the fact that he is blind, which is so often overlooked. From the moment Charlie enters the hospital for each visit, he is so vigilant. It is as if he fears that everyone is going to do something to him every time. His blindness creates an almost paranoid-like reaction in him.

Keren's training enables her to intuitively adapt her nonverbal behaviors to attune to Charlie. She does this by first suggesting that all go outside to the big lawn on the hospital campus. She chooses this approach on account of Charlie's blindness, thinking his olfactory senses may be enhanced outside, where he might be able to smell flowers in the garden, the lawn, and fresh air, in contrast with the smells in the hospital. This greatly contributes to his ability to calm down.

They sit on the lawn, and Keren tells him again that she is not going to go close to him or touch him, but rather is going to play with him.

DOI: 10.4324/9781003134800-7

She takes out two miniature plastic kidneys that she got from the nephrologist's office. Initially, Charlie remains vigilant and holds his body stiffly, but when she puts the kidneys in his hand, he starts to play with them. Keren says, "We have two things like this in our body and they help us pee. Your kidneys aren't working well and need to be repaired." She adds, "Your kidneys want food. This is why Mommy and Daddy want so much for you to eat." As Keren explains this, Charlie becomes more relaxed, softening his shoulders, freely moving them as he plays with the toy kidneys.

This case illustrates the therapeutic power of words and play for a very young child. Working through this case from a DMT perspective, we would add the observation of the sensory systems Charlie is using to engage with his environment, and which ones are the most sensitive. Tortora would also slow her own pace, making sure her nonverbal signals are calm. In particular, she makes sure her breathing is regulated and her voice is gentle yet audible. She is very purposeful and attentive to where she places her body in relationship to the child, watching carefully for any changes the child makes in his body, such as breathing more quickly, turning away, or gazing off. She would use this information to determine how close she can go to him.

Introduction

Being admitted to a hospital means a serious disruption in one's life, regardless of age. Children are particularly prone to the adverse impact of serious medical illness because, for them, the hospital can be like a foreign country where they are lost, feel intimidated, and are uncomfortable. Family environment and support has been found to be the strongest predictor of the outcome for children with medical illness (Goldberg et al., 1997). This result is in line with the fact that the younger the child, the greater his dependence on caregivers, while his limited verbal and cognitive skills put him at higher risk for having a very traumatic hospital experience. Although significant improvements in medical care have led to reduced mortality rates following critical illness, psychological sequelae have been shown to be meaningful (Davydow et al., 2008), as we will describe in this chapter in more detail. The American Academy of Pediatrics (Pediatrics, 2000) quote that says the goal of palliative care is "to add life to the child's years, not simply years to the child's life" reflects the huge changes in approaching pediatric care and hospitalization in the second half of the 20th century.

This chapter discusses how hospitals and medical teams have historically tried to address the quality of life for a baby with a life-threatening medical illness and the family. It highlights the importance of the presence of family members, and how and when this became a standard part of the child's hospital experience. We also review in this chapter the impact of long and/or recurrent hospitalizations for severe medical illnesses in general, and more specifically for pediatric cancer. There are very few studies that have focused on the critically ill infant's reactions to hospitalization.

Historical Review: The Gradual Understanding of the Impact of Hospitalization on Young Children

Until the late 1940s, it was widely accepted that it was undesirable for children in the hospital to be visited regularly by their parents. Many hospitals permitted monthly visitations only, and some not at all. During the 1950s, however, as the concept of separation anxiety became better known, there was growing concern about leaving young children in the hospital apart from their parents. This related to psychological theories about the importance of attachment. Rene Spitz (Spitz & Wolf, 1946), in England, described the clinical syndrome of "anaclitic depression," a term he used for babies who wasted away in hospitals due to the lack of development of an attachment relationship to any caregiver. In 1953, the Bow Arrow Hospital for children with tuberculosis in Dartford, England, took an innovative approach: Bed rest was an important component of tuberculosis treatment plans throughout the 1940s and 1950s, but the Bow Arrow team emphasized the role of play, alongside rest, in the process of the children's recovery. The hospital was physically set up to support this approach, featuring orderly rooms, as in a standard hospital, that were also child-friendly: There were children's toys, pictures on the walls, a piano and tables in the middle of the room, and the nursing staff were committed to facilitating playful, interpersonal interactions among the children during daily hospital life.

The first change in pediatric hospitalizations was to the physical environment. It took many years to understand the paramount importance of parents' presence at the hospital. It was not until the 1970s that unrestricted visiting became standard policy in U.S. public pediatric hospitals. In parallel, an organization named Child Life was created in the 1920s in the United States, aiming to improve hospital health care experiences for children by providing play and educational programs. The child life specialist became an early and ardent advocate for frequent family visits and parental participation in the child's care. This progressive philosophy was the precursor of family-centered care in hospitals.

In 1965, a group of women in health care met in Boston to share their work, their triumphs, and their challenges. The goal was to create child- and family-friendly hospital environments. They established in 1967 an association known as the Association for the Care of Children in Hospitals, renamed in 1979 as the Association for the Care of Children's Health.

ACCH membership included doctors, nurses, child life specialists, parents, and other health professionals working with children and families. During the 1970s, the number of child life programs increased substantially, and colleges developed academic curricula that incorporated hospital internships to prepare students to work with hospitalized children. A method of professional certification was adopted that assured a standard of practice for child life specialists, and by 1998 a standardized child life professional certification examination had been put in place. Today, child life professionals work and influence the delivery of care in health care and community settings. Certified child life specialists work in pediatric inpatient units, including critical care units, and in outpatient areas, including emergency departments, radiology and imaging, specialty-care clinics, and behavioral and rehabilitation facilities. They also work in community outreach programs, private practice, hospice services, home health, camps for children with health care needs, private medical and dental practices, and services for children of adult patients. Child life specialists continue to help infants, children, youth, and families cope with the stress and uncertainty of illness, injury, and treatment. This initiative, which started in children's hospitals in the United States, was replicated in many other Western countries. The creation of pediatric hospitals, rather than just having pediatric departments within hospitals for adults, has been an additional development that reflects a deeper understanding of the importance of the hospital setting in shaping the emotional outcome for the child with medical illness.

Children's Emotional Reactions to Hospitalization Due to Chronic Illness

Children vary in their capacities to cope with the stress of hospitalization. To accommodate them, many changes have been implemented in pediatric hospitals worldwide, with an increased awareness of the need to go beyond the narrow focus on medical aspects of pediatric illness to provide age-appropriate communication, support, and empathy from the medical and psychological staff. Even with improvements in early detection of those in distress, a significant number of children still suffer from some degree of emotional distress due to their medical experience. Estimates of the incidence of emotional problems resulting from hospital experience vary from 10–30 percent for severe psychological distress (continuing anxiety, separation anxiety, sleep problems, irritability, and aggressiveness), to as much as 90 percent for slight emotional upset (Rokach, 2016). Prolonged and repeated hospitalization increases the chance of later problems, as the children fall behind in their normal routines and activities, lose school time and contact with peers, and are less involved in family activities.

During admission, the separation of the child from familiar figures may be the cause of some of the emotional upset. Hospitalized children are often in a state of waiting and increased vigilance. Being confined to bed may be perceived by the child as a punishment and an endless state of imprisonment, regardless of the actual length of stay at the hospital (Rokach, 2016). Individual factors such as the children's temperament and intelligence contribute to their style of coping and may influence the short-term and long-term effects of hospitalization. Children who take an active coping role and are more cooperative with hospital staff are less disturbed after discharge. Thus, preparing children for the experience of hospitalization is very effective in reducing their emotional distress during admission.

It is important to reiterate that the stress these children endure is simultaneously physical and emotional. The attachment system is very much activated whenever the young child feels scared, tired, and in pain. In usual circumstances, physical closeness to the caregiver is what helps her, but confinement to the hospital, and sometimes isolation because of immune deficiencies, make her feel lonely and scared, especially when the attachment figures are themselves anxious and unable to calmly respond to the child. Young children often react more to being away from home and siblings than to the illness itself, and often interpret hospitalization as punishment for something they have done wrong (Rokach, 2016). It is very difficult for young children to understand that injections, blood tests, and transfusions are actually for the purpose of making them feel better in the long run. This fear may lead to strong resistance to subsequent medical procedures. At the hospital, the children's level of physical activity is inherently limited, and their play is often characterized by repetitive, solitary themes, instead of being a means for coping.

Critical illness leads to a cascade of physiological changes, in addition to the impact of the hospitalization itself, as previously described. Too low or too high cortisol levels have been observed in children (and adults) during severe physiological stress, plus links between cortisol, illness severity, and poor physical outcome (Joosten et al., 2000). Activation of the hypothalamic–pituitary–adrenal (HPA) axis is required for normal functioning, but excessive stimulation in various situations such as critical physical illness, traumatic injuries, and child maltreatment, may lead to subsequent and persistent anomalies in the regulation of the axis. The psychological sequelae of pediatric critical illness may be linked with these anomalies, as shown in a study (Als et al., 2017) that looked at the diurnal variation in basal salivary cortisol in 5–16-year-olds and children 3–6 months post-discharge and in healthy controls. Physically, the children felt better, but psychological sequelae were already apparent. The results showed a significant positive correlation between symptoms of PTSD and high pre-bedtime cortisol levels, but the authors could not rule out a premorbid cortisol dysregulation and a predisposition to developing PTSD symptoms.

In spite of increased awareness about the potentially detrimental impact of hospitalizations on the child's biosocioemotional development, there is still a relative lack of specific attention to the infancy age range, even though younger children, especially those between 6 months old and 4 years old, are the most vulnerable because of their limited cognitive and verbal abilities to work through negative feelings and understand the whole situation. The impact of the chronic severe illness itself and of the hospitalization experience on the young child and the parents need to be differentiated, as the hospitalization may be more frightening to the child than being at home while sick. Some parents may have the opposite experience: They may feel safer when the responsibility for the child's medical care is on the team. But for others, the loss of control over the child's care and the need to trust the medical staff make hospitalization extremely distressing. These situations may impinge on the parental relationship, especially if the co-parenting alliance (McHale & Lindahl, 2011) was fragile before the child's illness.

The younger the child is, the more dependent he is on the quality of his caregivers' co-parenting skills; therefore, it is of paramount importance to detect families at risk. Infants may develop symptoms of PTSD, as defined in the DC: 0–5™ (Zero To Three, 2016). The risk factors for an infant to develop PTSD symptoms have been identified as follows: the father's past history of PTSD, the mother's self-perception as unable to protect her child, a difficult child's temperament, poor family functioning, and lack of support. Parental distress reactions to their child's life-threatening illness are also risk factors for PTSD in the child (Landolt et al., 2012; Muscara et al., 2015). Protective factors include physical proximity of the infant to a secure attachment figure, parental adaptive mechanisms for coping with stress, cooperative co-parenting, and the infant's adequate developmental skills.

At the Pediatric Intensive Care Unit

Even with the overall effort to improve the pediatric hospital setting, being in a pediatric intensive care unit (PICU) has been linked with increased risk of significant and persistent emotional and behavioral problems. Approximately 25 percent of children exhibit maladaptive behaviors within the first year post-discharge (Carnevale, 1997; Colville 2008; Rees et al., 2004; Rennick et al., 2014; Rennick & Rashotte, 2009; Als et al., 2015), including poor self-esteem, anxiety, sleep disturbances, social isolation, symptoms of PTSD, and major depression (Davydow et al., 2008). This is not surprising, given that critical illness exposes children and their parents to extreme stressors such as highly invasive procedures, separation from the family, exposure to other critically ill children, continuous exposure to high levels of light and noise, and encounters with many caretaking strangers. A distinction needs to be made among injury-related traumatic events, illness-related traumatic events, and treatment-related traumatic events (Ward-Begnoche, 2007). Retrospective studies of school-age children demonstrated distortion in their recall of medical procedure events, endotracheal intubation, and pain (Colville, 2008).

Children under age 6 years, the majority of the PICU population, have not systematically been included in research. Preschoolers are usually excluded from studies because they are more difficult to assess and there is a lack of validated instruments. One exception, though, is the study in which children who were younger, more severely ill, and who endured more invasive procedures had significantly greater medical fears, a lower sense of control over their health, and ongoing post-traumatic stress responses for six months post-discharge (Rennick et al., 2014). Their findings indicate that regardless of the quality of the hospital setting, invasiveness plus length of stay and severity of illness in young children may have adverse long-term effects. Furthermore, the impact of the PICU hospitalization on the psychosocial well-being of all family members was shown in their follow-up study one year post-discharge (Rennick et al., 2021). Four major themes were identified: processing PICU reminders and memories, changes in perceptions of health and illness, changes in sense of self, and altered family dynamics due to long absences and new or changed caregiving roles. Increased vigilance and concern were observed in parents and siblings, highlighting the importance of long-term follow-up care that is aimed at supporting the whole family's psychological recovery.

The Impact of Specific Life-Threatening Medical Entities

With *heart disease* and *cystic fibrosis*, the diagnosis of an infant's congenital abnormality is especially stressful for parents. Parenting stress has been observed in one out of five parents of children from age 2–12 years, regardless of the severity of the child's cardiac status. This was especially observable in their difficulty with setting limits for their child (Uzark & Jones, 2003).

An innovative longitudinal study (Goldberg et al., 1990) of 28 infants with cystic fibrosis and 23 infants with congenital heart disease (CHD), compared with 33 healthy infants, looked at the 12- and 18-month-old infants' attachment patterns to their mothers, and the level of the child's autonomy/dependence at age 2. The healthy group included the highest proportion of securely attached infants, and those with CHD included the lowest. At 2 years, the healthy children had the most positive parent–infant relationship. Still, among the infants with medical illness, the link between secure attachment and positive interaction at age 2 was not found, in contrast with the healthy group where, as predicted, secure infants had a more positive interaction than insecure ones. These results brought attention to the important fact that severe and chronic medical illness may alter the protective function of secure attachment in the parent–infant relationship.

A more recent study on infants with cystic fibrosis (Tluczek et al., 2015) has shown an inverse correlation between parental perception of child vulnerability and the quality of the parent–infant interaction. High parental negative affect and/or inconsistent and intrusive behavior were associated with infant dysregulation and irritability. Congenital cardiomyopathies have been linked with numerous psychological problems in school-age children and adolescents, including inhibition of emotions, marked anxiety, depressive reaction, loneliness, low self-esteem, low body image, and emotional lability (Masi & Brovedani, 1996).

Finally, a very recent systematic review (Clancy et al., 2020) of 28 studies related to the impact of CHD on infant and young children's psychosocial development clearly showed a high prevalence of low-severity emotional and behavioral dysregulation. Young children with severe CHD manifested high rates of externalizing and internalizing symptoms and poor social development.

Accidental *burns* are quite common among children younger than 5 years old. Still, there is only scarce data available on the psychological impact of burns on the infant and very young child. A qualitative study of the aftermath of burn injury (Egberts et al., 2018) from eight children's perspectives identified three main categories of themes: vivid memories of the accident, the importance of parental support, and psychosocial impact of the burn injury and coping with it. The authors emphasized the importance of collecting and listening to the children's appraisals. With infants, even though they are unable to verbally express their experience of the burn injury, they may have vivid and frightening memories, which are often triggered by distress-provoking reminders of the accident. Parents and medical staff must be aware of this so they can detect and contain the infant's distress in real time (De Young et al., 2016). Prevalence rates from 6.5–29 percent have been reported for acute stress reactions among very young children within the first month after a car accident or burn injury, and a full-blown PTSD rate of 10 percent six months after the burn accident. Highly co-morbid with PTSD were reports of depression, separation anxiety disorder, oppositional defiant disorders, and specific phobias (De Young et al., 2016).

Symptoms of PTSD have been reported in children with *cancer* and their parents (Phipps et al., 2005), especially among those who have been recently diagnosed. More specifically, in the situation of a life-threatening illness, a recent study (Graf et al., 2013) has assessed PTSD in 48 children with cancer, age 8–48 months, about 15 months after their diagnosis. The assessment was based on questionnaires completed by mothers and the attending pediatric oncologist: 18.8 percent met the criteria for full PTSD, and 41.7 percent for partial PTSD. An older child age at diagnosis and maternal PTSD severity were risk factors for full and partial PTSD. The authors suggest that a younger age might have served as a protective factor because the young children's limited cognitive and developmental skills shielded them from understanding the severity of their illness. Still, the finding might also reflect the limitations of assessing very young children. In keeping with this hypothesis, parameters related to illness severity did not significantly predict PTSD in this sample. Regarding maternal PTSD as a risk factor, symptomatic mothers may indeed have a limited capacity for providing a stress buffer for their young children (Stoddard et al., 2006).

Obviously, pediatric cancer – with its physical, psychological, socioeconomic, and behavioral effects on children and their caregivers – represents a huge challenge for the family (Toledano-Toledano & de la Rubia, 2018). Still, families that adapt to the diagnosis are proactive, gather information, search for resources, are sociable, find support networks, and cooperate with the medical team. Resilience to disease is a process of positive adaptation despite the loss of health, and involves the development of vitality and skills to overcome the adversity.

A measurement scale of parental resilience has recently been developed with five main factors: personal competence, self-confidence, secure relationships and acceptance of change, and self-control (Toledano-Toledano et al., 2019). The concept of dyadic coping (Ferraz de Arruda-Colli et al., 2018) is helpful in the detection of vulnerable caregivers who struggle to cope with their child's cancer. The interpersonal process of dyadic coping may be positive or negative: Positive dyadic coping refers to situations when one partner assists the other in her/his coping efforts, and may even become an opportunity for relationship growth; in negative dyadic coping, no mutual support is observed. To our best knowledge, no study has looked at the impact of the quality of parental dyadic coping on the infant's own ability to cope with illness. The available studies address the parents' psychological reactions to the diagnosis of cancer and the stressors they face through the treatment process, such as financial burdens, perceptions of life threat, intensity and invasiveness of treatment, and other negative life events. In a recent study of parent psychological distress after the diagnosis of cancer (Vernon et al., 2017), 41 mothers and 25 fathers of infants younger than 2 years old who either had a cancer diagnosis (n = 37; infant patients) or was an infant sibling of an older child with cancer (n = 29; infant siblings) were recruited from a single oncology center. Mothers (47.5 percent) and fathers (37.5 percent) reported elevated cancer-related, post-traumatic stress symptoms, while rates of depression (12.2 percent of mothers and 12.0 percent of fathers) and anxiety symptoms (17.1 percent of mothers and 8.0 percent of fathers) were lower. Parent anxiety was higher with increased time post-diagnosis. No demographic or illness-related variables were associated with psychological distress, with the exception of the number of children in the family. Another recent study (Muscara et al., 2017) investigated factors associated with acute stress symptoms in 115 mothers and 56 fathers of children with serious illness who were treated in oncology, cardiology, and intensive care departments of a pediatric hospital. They found that psychosocial factors explained 36.8 percent of the variance in parent stress responses, while demographics added another 4.5 percent, but illness-related factors did not contribute.

Sickle cell disease is still a significant chronic hereditary medical problem in some parts of the world, and the children's mental health functioning is often overlooked (Bakri et al., 2004). The disease is characterized by severe, unpredictable, and recurrent pain, accompanied by anemia and an increased frequency of anxiety, depression, withdrawal, low self-esteem, poor interpersonal relationships, neurocognitive impairments, and maladaptive coping behaviors (Hijmans et al., 2009). Seventy school-age children with this disease were compared with 67 healthy children, and showed a high frequency of internalizing problems in the clinical range and less total competence (Trzepacz et al., 2004). The overall impact of the disease among children 1.5–5 years old (n = 35) as compared with a control group of healthy children at a vaccination clinic (n = 35) showed an increased level of internalizing symptoms (emotional lability, anxiety, depression, somatic complaints), as well as externalizing ones (aggression, especially) and sleep problems (Bakri et al., 2004). As mentioned in Chapter 5, sustained withdrawal is a common reaction in infants with chronic pain. Bakri's study is one of the few that have addressed the age range of toddlerhood and is therefore important, despite its small sample size.

When Risk Factors Cluster Together

The following vignette illustrates the complex processes parents and child experience, together and individually, while facing a very early and continuous life-threatening condition.

> Olive, 1 year, 9 months old, is referred to Keren by the hospital gastroenterologist who is trying to wean her off gastrostomy feeding. Olive is the only child of her parent couple and was the fruit of an IVF pregnancy, but she has a half-sister, a teenager from her father's first marriage. On day four after birth, Olive started vomiting, and on day eight, she was diagnosed with Alagille syndrome, pulmonic stenosis, and kidney dysfunction.
>
> Alagille syndrome is a congenital syndrome, due to chromosome 20p abnormality, that includes arterio-hepatic dysplasia; characteristic facies (prominent forehead and nasal bridge, eyes set deep and apart, small chin, prominent ears), jaundice due to direct hyperbilirubinemia, persistent pruritus starting at from 3–6 months, cardiovascular

abnormalities, vertebral arch defects, and dysplastic kidneys. Some 30–40 percent of children with Alagille's need liver transplantation because of severe cholestasis.

Olive stays at the hospital during her whole first year of life because she has unexplained fever and recurrent vomiting, and Mother is afraid to take her home. A nasogastric tube is inserted, followed by gastrostomy at 10 months, because, for an unclear reason, Olive stopped eating and would only drink. In parallel, she also developed breath-holding spells, and the parents did everything they could to prevent her from crying.

Olive's parents have a chronically stormy relationship that remains so after unsuccessful couples therapy. Both parents have been diagnosed with borderline personality disorder. Mother creates strong antagonism among the medical staff (lack of trust, very demanding threats of lawsuits, etc.). Olive, who has not yet entered day care because of her unstable medical condition and fear of intercurrent infections, has very limited social contacts.

Both parents and Olive are present during my first meeting with them as the child psychiatrist. The parents' immediate concern is Olive's breath-holding spells, which frighten them. Olive is also becoming tyrannical at home, though very compliant with medications and gastrostomy feedings. In short, Olive is controlling her parents. This may be in response to her parents' control over her body and to their verbally abusive interpersonal communication. In any case, illness frightens the three of them. Fear for the child's life and anger fill the air.

After a few minutes together, a revealing micro-interactional event takes place: Olive steps heavily on her mother's foot. Mother does not react, though obviously in pain. I ask why she lets her do this, and Mother answers: "We allow her everything, never frustrate her, do everything for her . . . . She just has to stay alive . . . . For us, limit-setting and education are not relevant."

The medical team is caught within strong counter-transferential reactions, ambivalence, fear of failing the medical challenge, difficulty dealing with the parents, and empathy and compassion toward Olive. The severity of the young child's condition makes parents and staff put aside the emotional aspects of the situation. The case has been referred to psychiatry to address these emotional needs and support the medical team in dealing with their angry feelings toward the parents.

Together with the medical team and the parents, we decide to postpone weaning from gastrostomy until more basic goals are achieved, such as: "speaking the illness" with Olive ("What do you mean?" Mother replies. "She's not even 2 years old!"); making the parents understand their child's developmental needs of autonomy, individuation, and regulation; decreasing parental anxiety; letting the child start day care; and trying to improve the familial situation.

Two months after starting this therapeutic process, some improvements emerge: Olive enters day care easily, with no separation problems. She starts saying "no" and "me," and her breath-holding spells almost disappear. Olive starts to actively resist the gastrostomy feedings, trying to pull the peg out. The parents begin to realize their child's need to develop an image of her sick body, and I suggest they talk about how to make Olive's yellow skin tone and scratching feeling go away.

When Olive is approximately 28 months, Mother dares to leave her with Father, for the first time since Olive's birth. In Mother's absence, Olive takes food in her mouth – another first – and says, "I want to eat with my mouth." But Olive's jaundice deepens, and three months later, the team decides to have the liver and possibly kidney transplantation done abroad, which interrupts the weaning process. It takes several months to organize the travel. "To have the yellow go away" is what we all say during our last session before Olive and Mother leave the country.

Olive is now 3.5 years old. Before leaving home for the operation, she asks her half-sister, "If I eat well, and don't scratch myself, will I not have to go abroad?" The half-sister dares to ask her what frightens her . . . and she is able to answer, ". . . dying!" Her parents cannot believe Olive knows that word.

Olive undergoes the liver and kidney transplant operations and stays in the hospital abroad for a year and a half because of various complications. She gets weaned from gastrostomy and is toilet trained. Email back and forth between Mother and me act as a "secure word envelope" for the child via Mother, until they come back. Soon after their return, the renormalization process is interrupted again, this time by a transient ischemic attack, which requires the dangerous procedure of brain angiography. Dread is again present, but Olive has learned to put it in words. Just before the angiography, Olive tells the nurse, "I don't want the anesthesia . . . . I'm afraid not to wake up, not to talk . . . .". But the procedure is successful, and Olive is discharged. We continue to follow her, and the overall goals are achieved. Her parents resume their therapy.

Clinical Discussion

This case illustrates the interplay of risk factors in a severely medically compromised infant and her caregiving environment. Keren helps Olive find words for the felt experience of her body and her illness. Talking the illness to a very young child requires using simple words to concretely describe the illness, making a link between the treatment and illness. Olive doesn't know what it means to have a liver transplant; what she sees is her yellow skin, and what she feels is the itchiness. By explaining the goal of the operation as "to have the yellow skin and the scratchy feeling go away," Keren concretely addresses Olive's experience. The parents are wordless because they are paralyzed by fear of losing Olive, and because she is so young, they don't think she can understand. They needed Keren to be the translator.

The treatment creates a safe place for the parents and Olive to express their fears and worries. Strikingly, the parents are so overwhelmed by their fear of losing their child that they put aside the importance of setting limits and expecting the child to mature and become independent. They are also avoidant of their child's fearful emotions about her illness. Olive feels more confident telling her half-sister – not her parents – about her fear of not waking up from the anesthesia. Keren facilitates a way for Olive to speak about her difficult feelings by simply discussing them rather than avoiding her fears.

Keren states, "I work with many children here at the hospital, and all of them are afraid." Lieberman's principles of Child-Parent Psychotherapy (CPP) in traumatic situations (Lieberman & Van Horn, 2008) are very useful in translating the meaning of the young child's behavior for the parent and vice versa, and to link them with the traumatic experiences they have been living. The process is based on the assumption that both parents and their young child sense danger but are afraid talking about it will make it bigger. Putting feelings into words is the main role of the CPP trauma-oriented therapist.

Conclusion

Pediatric medical care has come a long way since the time when parents were not allowed to stay at the hospital with their infants with medical conditions. But there is still a tendency to minimize the extent to which the very young child perceives the severity of her condition, her parents' dread, and the medical staff's emotional reactions. Although there are commonalities in how life-threatening illnesses impact the young child's socioemotional development, there are also distinct influences from specific illnesses on the infant's and the parents' perceptions. The explanation for this differential impact is not always obvious. For instance, it is unclear why congenital heart failure has a more adverse impact than cystic fibrosis. Hence, for each case, one has to assess the parents' perception of the specific disease, the impact of its symptoms on the infant (infants are often more disturbed by painful symptoms less significant in terms of prognosis than by the disease itself), and the nature of the medical procedures. This must all be taken within the context of the parents' strengths and weaknesses, support sources, and cultural beliefs.

As illustrated throughout this book, we suggest these very complex situations are best handled by the complementary work of a dance/movement therapy approach, along with child psychiatry, with the aims of soothing the infant and the parents by putting words to painful and frightening procedures and feelings into words, facilitating embodied play, supporting the parents in their parenting functions, and promoting their child's development. No less important is the work with the medical team, teaching them about what and how infants perceive, understand, and react, facilitating and often mediating communication between them and the parents.

References

Als, L., Picouto, M., Hau, S., Nadel, S., Cooper, M., Pierce, C., Kramer, T., & Garralda, M. (2015). Mental and physical well-being following admission to pediatric intensive care. *Pediatric Critical Care Medicine, 16*, 141–149.

Als, L., Picouto, M., O'Donnell, K., Nadel, S., Cooper, M., & Pierce, C. (2017). Stress hormones and post traumatic stress symptoms following pediatric critical illness: An exploratory study. *European Child and Adolescent Psychiatry, 26*, 511–519.

Bakri, M., Ismail, E., Elsedfy, G., Amr, M., & Ibrahim, A. (2004). Behavioral impact of sickle cell disease in young children with repeated hospitalization. *Paediatric Anaesthesia, 14*, 910–915.

Carnevale, F. (1997). The experience of critically ill children: Narratives of unmaking. *Intensive Critical Care Nursing, 13*, 49–52.

Clancy, T., Jordan, B., de Weeth, C., & Muscara, F. (2020). Early emotional behavioral and social development of infants and young children with congenital heart disease: A systematic review. *Journal of Clinical Psychology in Medical Settings, 27*(4), 686–703. https://doi.org/10.1007/s10880-019-09651-1.

Colville, G. (2008). The psychological impact on children of admission to intensive care. *Pediatrics Clinics of North America, 55*, 605–616.

Davydow, D., Richardson, L., Zatzick, D., & Katon, W. (2008). Psychiatric morbidity in pediatric critical illness survivors: A comprehensive review of the literature. *Archives of Pediatric and Adolescent Medicine, 164*, 377–385.

De Young, A., Ac, H., Kenardy, J., Kimble, R., & Landolt, M. (2016). Coping with accident reactions (CARE) early intervention programme for preventing traumatic stress reactions in young injured children: Study protocol for two randomized controlled trials. *Trials, 17*, 362.

Egberts, M., Geenen, R., de Jong, A., Hofland, H., & Van Loey, N. (2018, September 29). The aftermath of burn injury from the child's perspective: A qualitative study. *Journal of Health and Psychology.* doi:135910531880826.

Ferraz de Arruda-Colli, M., Bedoya, S., Muriel, A., Pelletier, W., & Wiener, L. (2018). In good times and in bad: What strengthens or challenges a parental relationship during a child's cancer trajectory? *Journal of Psychosocial Oncology, 36*, 635–648.

Goldberg, S., Janus, M., Washington, J., Simmons, R., Maclusky, I., & Fowler, R. (1997). Prediction of preschool behavioral problems in healthy and pediatric samples. *Journal of Development and Behavioral Pediatrics, 18*, 304–313.

Goldberg, S., Washington, J., Morris, P., Fischer-Fay, A., & Simmons, R. (1990). Early diagnosed chronic illness and mother-child relationships in the first two years. *Canadian Journal of Psychiatry, 35*, 726–733.

Graf, A., Bergstraesser, E., & Landolt, M. (2013). Posttraumatic stress in infants and pre-schoolers with cancer. *Psycho-Oncology, 22*, 1543–1548.

Hijmans, C., Grootenhuis, M., Oosterlaan, J., Last, B., Heijboer, H., Peters, M., et al. (2009). Behavioral and emotional problems in children with sickle cell disease and healthy siblings: Multiple informants, multiple measures. *Pediatric Blood Cancer, 53*, 1277–1283.

Joosten, K., De Kleijn, E., Westerterp, M., De Hoog, M., Eijick, F., & Hop, W. (2000). Endocrine and metabolic responses in children with meningococcal sepsis: Striking differences between survivors and non survivors. *Journal of Clinical Endocrinology and Metabolism, 85*, 3746–3753.

Landolt, M., Ystrom, E., Sennhauser, F., Gnehm, H., & Vollrath, M. (2012). The mutual prospective influence of child and parental post traumatic stress symptoms in pediatric patients. *Journal of Child Psychology and Psychiatry, 53*, 767–774.

Lieberman, A., & Van Horn, P. (2008). *Psychotherapy with infants and young children: Reparing the effects of stress and trauma on early attachment.* The Guilford Press.

Masi, G., & Brovedani, P. (1996). Psychopathology of chronic diseases in children and adolescents: Congenital cardiopathies. *Minerva Cardiangiology, 44*, 479–493.

McHale, J., & Lindahl, K. (2011). *Coparenting: A conceptual and clinical examination of family systems.* American Psychological Association.

Muscara, F., McCarthy, M., Thompson, E., Heanaey, C., & Hearps, S. (2017). Psychosocial, demographic, and illness-related factors associated with acute traumatic stress responses in parents of children with serious illness or injury. *Journal of Trauma and Stress, 30*, 237–244.

Muscara, F., McCarthy, M., Woolf, C., Hearps, S., Burke, K., & Anderson, V. (2015). Early psychological reactions in parents of children with a life threatening illness within a pediatric hospital setting. *European Psychiatry, 30*, 555–561.

Pediatrics, A. A. O. (2000). Committee on bioethics and committee on hospital care. *Pediatrics, 106*, 353.

Phipps, S., Long, A., Hudson, M., & Rai, S. (2005). Symptoms of post traumatic stress in children with cancer and their parents: Effects of informant and time from diagnosis. *Pediatric Blood Cancer, 45*, 952–959.

Rees, G., Gledhill, J., Garralda, M., & Nadel, S. (2004). Psychiatric outcome following pediatric intensive care unit (PICU admission: A cohort study). *Intensive Care Medicine, 30*, 1607–1614.

Rennick, J., Dougherty, G., Chambers, C., Stremier, R., Childerhose, J., et al. (2014). Children's psychological and behavioral responses following pediatric intensive care unit hospitalization: The caring intensively study. *BMC Pediatrics, 14*.

Rennick, J., Knox, A., Treherne, S., Dryden-Palmer, K., Stremler, R., et al. (2021). Family members' perceptions of their psychological responses one year following pediatric intensive care unit (PICU) hospitalisation: Qualitative findings from the caring intensely study. *Frontiers in Pediatrics, 9*, 1–11.

Rennick, J., & Rashotte, J. (2009). Psychological outcomes in children following pediatric intensive care unit hospitalization: A systematic review of the research. *Journal of Child Health Care, 13*, 128–149.

Rokach, A. (2016). Psychological, emotional and physical experiences of hospitalized children. *Clinical Case Reports and Review, 2*, 399–401.

Spitz, R., & Wolf, K. (1946). Anaclitic depression: An inquiry into the genesis of psychiatric conditions in early childhood. *Psychoanalytic Study of the Child, 2*, 313–342.

Stoddard, S. G., Ronfeldt, H., et al. (2006). Acute stress symptoms in young children with burns. *Journal of American Academy of Child and Adolescent Psychiatry*, *45*, 87–93.

Tluczek, A., Clark, R., McKechnie, A., & Brown, R. (2015). Factors affecting parent-child relationships one year after positive newborn screening for cystic fibrosis or congenital hypothyroidism. *Journal of Developmental and Behavioral Pediatrics*, *36*, 24–34.

Toledano-Toledano, F., & de la Rubia, J. (2018). Factors associated with anxiety in family caregivers of children with chronic diseases. *Biopsychosocial Medicine*, *12*.

Toledano-Toledano, F., de la Rubia, J., Broche-Perez, Y., Dominguez-Guedea, M., & Granados-Garcia, V. (2019). The measurement scale of resilience among family caregivers of children with cancer: A psychometric evaluation. *BMC Public Health*, *19*.

Trzepacz, A., Vannatta, K., Gerhrdt, C., Ramey, C., & Noll, R. (2004). Emotional, social, and behavioral functioning of children with sickle cell disease and comparison peers. *Journal of Pediatric Hematology and Oncology*, *26*, 642–648.

Uzark, K., & Jones, K. (2003). Parenting stress and children with heart disease. *Journal of Pediatric Health Care*, *17*, 163–168.

Vernon, L., Eyles, D., Hulbert, C., Bretherton, L., & McCarthy, M. (2017). Infancy and pediatric cancer: An exploratory study of parent psychological distress. *Psychooncology*, *26*, 361–368.

Ward-Begnoche, W. (2007). Post traumatic stress symptoms in the pediatric intensive care unit. *Journal of Specialized Pediatric Nursing*, *12*, 84–92.

Zero To Three. (2016). *Diagnostic classification of mental health and developmental disorders of infancy and early childhood: DC: 0–5.* Zero To Three Press.

Chapter 7

Long-Term Effects of Chronic Life-Threatening Pediatric Illness on Later Adjustment and Their Clinical Implications

A young mother comes to me (Keren) with her 3-year-old son for a consultation about his extreme selective eating. She expresses her frustration, as they have been in treatment at a "failure to thrive" outpatient clinic for two years with no results. She adds as a "by the way": "Anyway, I don't have much trust toward people and health systems." Reflecting on the possible origin for her general lack of trust, the mother reveals to me the medical traumatic experience she went though: Her eyes fill with tears while she tells me how, at age 14, she spent almost a year in the hospital because of a lymphoma that was diagnosed late, saying: "I had had symptoms for months before I was diagnosed, but my parents and the doctors thought I was faking being tired all the time. Since then, I have trouble trusting others, especially when it is about medical stuff."

Introduction

From this vignette we can learn how early medical experiences leave prominent traces on one's psyche, feeling associations that may become activated while parenting a very sick infant. This chapter reviews the role early medical experiences play in psychological functioning. Most of the longitudinal studies on the psychological impact of life-threatening illness in early childhood are about cancer, although uncertainty and pain are important factors that influence long-term psychological functioning, regardless of the type of illness (Szulczewski et al., 2017).

Today, nearly 90 percent of children diagnosed with cancer survive at least five years post-diagnosis, and more than 70 percent survive for ten years (Howlader et al., 2016). This is one of modern medicine's true successes, but there is not enough focus on how survivors of childhood cancer frequently experience delayed and long-term effects of the disease and its intensive treatment, including chronic pain and medical conditions, and cognitive, behavioral, and emotional impairments (Bitsko et al., 2016; Marcoux et al., 2016; Anderson & Kunin-Batson, 2009; Stein et al., 2008). These later effects are due not only to the damaging side effects of chemotherapy, cranial irradiation, and surgery, but also to the cancer-linked traumatic experiences the child and family endure. An Early Adversity

DOI: 10.4324/9781003134800-8

Framework has been developed and applied (Marusak et al., 2018) to understand the complex interplay between all the biological and psychological factors, and even more importantly, to plan for early therapeutic measures aimed at preventing at least some of the impairment.

We start this chapter by reviewing the long-term impact of life-threatening chronic illnesses with emphasis on embedded uncertainty and pain, then we focus on the neurodevelopmental and psychological impacts of pediatric cancer on survivors since most of the longitudinal studies have been performed in this patient population; but our approach to supporting families and their children can be applied to any early life-threatening illness. We close with a clinical vignette to illustrate how dance/movement therapy can be beneficial to the child and parents in the years after the acute phase of an illness.

Pain and Its Impact on Later Adjustment

Pain is a common experience among children with chronic severe illness, such as juvenile rheumatic diseases, inflammatory bowel disorders, and cancer. Up to 58.7 percent of pediatric cancer survivors report either acute pain (after a medical procedure or an acute illness), episodic pain (recurrent experiences of pain with in-between painless periods), or chronic pain (almost daily pain for at least three months) (Huang et al., 2013). Pain, which has been associated with elevated suicidal ideation and distress (Recklitis et al., 2010), is distressing in itself but also as a potentially threatening indicator of the recurrence of cancer or a treatment-related complication (Zebrack & Chesler, 2002). Survivors who experience significant pain show increased internalizing and externalizing symptoms (Brinkman et al., 2016).

Regardless of its origin, the experience of pain involves a complex interplay of neural pathways that are implicated in its physical and emotional aspects (Simons et al., 2014). For instance, the salience and emotional network (SEN) is very involved in pain expectation, perception, and distress. Impairments in attention, memory, and cognitive control have been demonstrated (Annett et al., 2015) among survivors of pediatric cancer, with impacts on the survivors' ability to cope with pain by controlling and shifting their attention from the pain experience.

Several biological factors have been associated with increased rates of pain and poorer health-related quality of life, including types of cancer (e.g. osteosarcoma), cancer treatments (vincristine and platinum-based chemotherapy medications, central nervous system irradiation, and surgery), younger age at diagnosis, and female gender (Huang et al., 2013). These findings imply clinicians should be aware of the potential impact of pain experiences that may last beyond the effects of cancer or the life-threatening illness itself.

The Impact of Uncertainty in Pediatric Chronic Severe Illness

Illness uncertainty has been associated with psychological functioning and coping in studies among children with chronic illnesses and adults (Stewart & Mishel, 2000; Wright et al., 2009). Pediatric illness uncertainty experienced by the caregiver and the child requires consideration of the child's developmental level, the need to separately assess the caregiver's and the child's level of uncertainty, and the mutual impact of each of these on the other (Fedele et al., 2013).

Uncertainty about the child's illness has been associated with overall poor quality of life (Fortier et al., 2013) and psychosocial functioning (Carpentier et al., 2007), as well as increased anxiety and depression (Carpentier et al., 2007). Obviously, the influence of caregivers is of paramount importance, but only a few notable studies assess both the caregiver's and the child's reports of uncertainty and their reciprocal impact (Fedele et al., 2012; Page et al., 2012; Stewart et al., 2010). They find that caregiver uncertainty is not only associated with their own psychological functioning, but also with their child's. Additional research is needed to determine more precise mean effect sizes, as well as the potential efficacy of intervention to address uncertainty (Szulczewski et al., 2017).

Neurodevelopmental and Emotional Long-Term Consequences of Pediatric Cancer and Its Treatment

Cognitive, behavioral, and emotional impairments have been reported among some survivors of pediatric cancer (Cheung & Krull, 2015; Ashford et al., 2010). Cognitive dysfunction has been estimated to be as high as 67 percent for attentional deficits, and 3–28 percent for deficits in other cognitive domains, including executive functioning, IQ, memory, processing speed, and visual-motor integration (Castellino et al., 2014). Anxiety, depression, and PTSD have been reported in a subset of child survivors (McDonnell et al., 2017; Price et al., 2016; Oancea et al., 2014). In a very recent study (Tillery et al., 2019), caregivers of 50 children, age 3–6 years, with cancer and 47 healthy children completed diagnostic scales for the assessment of PTSD. Only three children in the patient group and none in the comparison group met criteria for PTSD. Still, other emotional or behavioral symptoms may be present.

Parental distress and child temperament were significantly correlated with post-traumatic stress symptoms. Regarding lifetime rates of PTSD among cancer survivors, the St. Jude Lifetime Cohort (Allen et al., 2018) found that most adult survivors do not identify cancer as their most stressful event, and report a non–cancer-related event as most traumatic;

only one in eight adult survivors of childhood cancer had PTSD symptoms above the cutoff. It is also important to note that cancer-related psychological issues may emerge insidiously years or even decades after the actual cancer occurrence, as do other forms of childhood adversity (Caspi et al., 2014).

The very experience of cancer in childhood constitutes a serious deviation from the expectable safe rearing environment, and in that sense, it should be conceptualized as an adverse childhood experience (ACE), regardless of the type of cancer (Marusak et al., 2018). Stress and adversity do not end after the child completes his cancer treatment. The transition to survivorship is no less challenging for the child and her family, as everyone needs to readjust to home, school, and peers, often while still experiencing physical limitations and chronic pain (Hobbie et al., 2010). Worries about health and risk of recurrence require ongoing medical monitoring, which in itself engenders hypervigilance and anxiety, impinging on the child and family functioning.

The majority (60 percent) of existing studies on the impact of childhood cancer have been in patients with central nervous system tumors, the second most common pediatric cancer. For instance, acute lymphoblastic leukemia (ALL), the most common type of pediatric cancer and a non-CNS cancer, is now treated with chemotherapy rather than cranial irradiation, and yet significant cognitive, behavioral, and emotional late effects have been reported (Trentacosta et al., 2016; Cheung & Krull, 2015). Marusak's model views cancer treatment (including variables of modality, intensity, dosage, and duration), together with early threat exposure (life-threatening disease, invasive medical interventions, threat to physical integrity, and disability), as the two main factors that imprint on brain development and determine the range of cognitive, behavioral, and emotional late and long-term effects of pediatric cancer, regardless of its type. Their impact is mediated by external risk and protective factors (education, family functioning, community resources, nutrition, physical activity, peer interactions, and support), as well as individual differences (including genes, temperament, age, developmental stage, and gender).

The hippocampus and the SEN regions in the brain seem to be especially sensitive to pediatric cancer. The SEN is involved in a wide range of cognitive and affective functions, as it detects and orients attention to biologically or cognitively relevant internal and external stimuli (Seeley et al., 2007). The ability to interpret, regulate, and respond appropriately to social cues relies on the hippocampus and the SEN, so distorted perception of threat and safety may impinge on the child's ability to learn and interact with others in social circumstances. The hippocampus is sensitive to the neurotoxic effects of chemotherapy and radiation therapy, but also to the neurotoxic effects of exposure to threats during sensitive periods of brain development, i.e. the first years of life (Heim & Binder, 2012), as the hippocampus is one of the few brain areas that shows active postnatal neurogenesis (Kohman & Rhodes, 2013). In terms of "psychological toxicity," it is the unpredictable and uncontrollable course of cancer treatment, with its intrusive, unfamiliar, often painful medical procedures, that engenders overwhelming helplessness in the child and his family. As many as 75 percent of young adult survivors of childhood cancer report re-experiencing traumatic cancer-related events, and nearly 50 percent report increased physiological responses while remembering cancer (Price et al., 2016). The Childhood Cancer Survivor Study (CCSS) compares the outcomes of adult survivors of childhood cancer with those of a matched cohort of adult siblings and a population cohort (Zeltzer et al., 2009), looking at the impacts of various types of childhood cancer. Their main findings are that fatigue and psychological distress, including depression and anxiety, are significant in a subgroup of adult survivors, especially among women, unemployed, low SES, and those who suffer from late or delayed effects of cancer therapy.

Clinical Implications for Prevention of Long-Term Neurodevelopmental and Psychological Complications

Most individual survivors can expect a positive psychosocial adjustment in adulthood, but many survivors may continue to suffer psychological distress (Zeltzer et al., 2009). Ideally, late psychological effects are best prevented during the acute stage of cancer treatment in childhood. Research into the neurodevelopmental and psychological long-term consequences of pediatric cancer should be translated into early intervention during and after the acute phase of treatment. Existing public health prevention models have already been adapted to psychosocial screening and intervention in pediatric cancer at the universal, selected, and clinical levels. As we have reviewed previously, Maruzak's recent and comprehensive model adds the neurodevelopmental component to the psychological one, and is based on mapping each child's external and individual factors that will mediate the impact of exposure to a life threat and treatment. Early identification and treatment of this subgroup of children, even during the acute phase of cancer treatment, may be of paramount importance in preventing poor long-term adjustment outcomes. With many oncology teams, including Tortora's, mindfulness-based stress reduction (MBSR), dance/movement therapy, music therapy, yoga and other body–mind therapies, and cognitive therapies are introduced early in treatment as part of the standard of care.

Special attention should be paid to pain in cancer survivors. Historically, pain in children with cancer has been a focus of management during afflictive procedures and acute neuropathic pain. As we described previously, recent data show that pain is an ongoing concern for many survivors of pediatric cancer and requires the development of preventive models for this kind of care. An assessment and interdisciplinary intervention aimed at preventing and reducing pain, its related distress, and functional impairment was developed by using acute pain medications, child-life intervention, relaxation strategies, physical medicine, and rehabilitation during and after the acute phase of treatment (Stone et al., 2018).

In Tortora's clinical experience, many pediatric cancer survivors returning for annual follow-up visits fondly share memories of their therapeutic play with Tortora and her DMT colleagues. The use of multisensory dance/movement therapy (MSDMT) activities (see Chapter 11) for pain management during treatments enables them to reminisce about their playful experience without making an association to pain. Given the risk for persistent pain, Stone and colleagues recommend a routine screening for all survivors of pediatric cancer (i.e. universal level of prevention) using existing tools, such as Pediatric Pain Screening (PPST) (Simons et al., 2015) or the Pain Intensity and Pain Interference scales (PROMIS) (Stone et al., 2016). The younger the child, the stronger the emphasis should be on efforts to lower the parents' catastrophic reactions to the child's pain, which can exacerbate the child's own anxiety.

For those survivors with high-intensity and frequent pain, a targeted level of intervention is needed, meaning active support and monitoring with the aim of preventing the pain escalation, functional impairment, and affective distress. In-person or internet-delivered pain education programs can reinforce adaptive pain coping strategies (Robins et al., 2016), as well as cognitive bias modification (Lichtenthal et al., 2017). For those with pain-related daily impairment, a clinical level of intervention is required, and the recommended approach is to have an interdisciplinary cancer-related pain treatment team, similar to existing interdisciplinary teams for patients with chronic noncancer pain (Stahlschmidt et al., 2016).

Family Functioning and Parental Support

One cannot underestimate the importance of addressing family functioning in any preventive intervention for a child's long-term adjustment. Not surprisingly, greater family cohesion, expressiveness, support, and lowered family conflict have been associated with better child adjustment outcomes (Van Schoors et al., 2017). Each caregiver's emotional and embodied experience of parenting their baby during illness must be considered. As the result of long-term impacts of life-threatening illness, chronic pain, repeated invasive procedures, and anxiety-provoking follow-up visits on parents and child, patients who have experienced medical illness in their early years may come to our psychological and psychiatric attention because of seemingly unrelated problems, including temper tantrums, social anxiety, poor engagement with peers, attentional and regulatory difficulties, learning difficulties, fears, anxiety, depression, obsessive-compulsive behaviors, developmental milestones such as self-care and toileting, eating disorders, difficulties with siblings, and issues related to family dynamics.

Shifting away from the continuous, vigilant state of tension parents maintain during their child's illness can be very difficult. Many caregivers are surprised that their relief and joy in experiencing a now-healthy child create new anxieties and parenting issues, including difficulties in setting limits and appropriate behavioral expectations. They often discuss their inability to relax with the belief that their child is well, and describe emotionally, physically, and/or socially "falling apart" post-treatment after they finally let down their guard. Helping parents listen, attune, and respond to their own nonverbal cues is illuminating and soothing. It provides an avenue toward healing memories and creating a healthy pathway forward. Helping them understand the emotional and embodied responses they experience but may not be able to articulate, as well as making links between the child's traumatic experiences and dysfunctional symptoms, is our ultimate goal as mental health clinicians.

Of course, helping parents reflect on their reactions takes time. Tortora's Embodied Parenting (EP) method, discussed in Chapter 4, also supports parents after their child's acute medical experience by helping them slow down, observe, and evaluate their own and their child's nonverbal communications as expressions of their experience. In this stage of treatment, similar to Child Parent Psychotherapy (Lieberman, 2021; Lieberman & Van Horn, 2008), there are sessions with family members present and separate sessions for the child and parents. In the parenting sessions, caregivers discuss their experience of the child's illness, and they gain insight into coping methods they and their child developed during treatment, reflecting on how these behaviors are currently manifesting. Core symptoms, behaviors, and themes that bring young children into treatment include tantrums; social anxiety, especially with adults; difficulty engaging with siblings and peers; attentional and regulatory challenges; learning differences; fears; general anxiety; depression; obsessive-compulsive behaviors; delays achieving developmental milestones such as self-care and toileting; eating disorders; and issues related to family dynamics.

Understanding the roles of suppression and reappraisal (Gross, 2013), two very common forms of emotion regulation (ER) used to down-regulate emotion, provides valuable insight into how behaviors during medical treatment may influence ensuing difficult behaviors and family dynamics. In suppression, a behavior-oriented form of ER, emotional expression is decreased when one is aroused emotionally. Affectively, a decrease in positive emotion also occurs, but it does not create a physiological decrease in negative emotion. There is an increase in sympathetic nervous system responses and activation in emotion-generative regions of the brain, including the amygdala. Cognitively, suppression results in poorer subsequent memory in laboratory research. In reappraisal, a cognitive form of

ER, thinking is used to alter the emotional response to a specific situation. This leads to a decreased negative and increased positive emotional experience. The sympathetic nervous system responses are either not affected or are decreased, and there is reduced activation of the emotion-generative regions of the brain, including the ventral striatum and amygdala. Laboratory research on memory has shown no impact or improvement in memory when reappraisal is used.

Suppression is a necessary regulatory coping behavior in response to a medical experience, but distinguishing when suppression is interfering with post-treatment healing is invaluable. With parents, this occurs by helping them become aware of the discrepancy between how the felt experience of their internal emotional state – which, initially, may register only unconsciously – is affecting their state of mind and outward behaviors. Gaining this awareness is key to understanding underlying dynamics with their child, because their inner emotions may be subtly revealed and read by their child through the nature of verbal and nonverbal communications. We approach this by helping them express their true emotions while sharing stories of their experiences. Working from the body–mind–emotional perspective, as the parent speaks, the DMT pays close attention to tonal shifts in their voice and facial, gestural, and postural changes that demonstrate tension and emotion. The therapist helps the caregiver slow down and pause to reflect on their experience in the moment. As the parents release the tension they have been holding emotionally and physically, spontaneous emotions are frequently shared, often for the first time, enabling them to make associations about how their anxious, fearful demeanor during their child's illness is affecting dynamics with their child now. This supports a reappraisal of their experience, connecting their felt experiences with their emotions, prompting the caregiver to acknowledge and alter their emotional responses when thinking about and discussing medical events and previous interactions with their child. These new perspectives often result in adjustments that quickly improve the family dynamics.

During DMT sessions with the young child post-illness, the reappraisal takes on an embodied nature as the child expresses and symbolically enacts emotional themes evocative of their medical experience. Healing occurs as the child becomes empowered in their now-able body through the storylines of their dance-play. When and if a connection develops between themes that come out of physical play and the child's medical experience, whether they remain on the implicit symbolic level or are revealed explicitly is directed by the child. Joint sessions with the parents and their child are conducted with sensitivity, for their nonverbal behaviors can inadvertently trigger each other. Thus, the timing and frequency of these joint sessions is case-specific, based on individual needs and a careful reappraisal of their skills.

Clinical Vignette

For children who have a medical condition in early infancy, the importance of continuity in working psychologically at the verbal and nonverbal levels is illustrated in the following vignette, which features Tortora's work with a child who is four years past severe medical illness. The vignette in Chapter 8 also provides an example of a DMT intervention after medical illness.

> Angie, age 4, zips past me as I open the door of my private dance/ movement psychotherapy studio to let her and Mom inside. Whew! I barely introduce myself to Mom before flying after Angie, who has already pulled the colorful scarves off their wall of hooks and is about to empty the cabinet shelf of its toys. As I approach, Angie takes off again, this time circling the room like it's a racetrack. She shoots me a bright smile, which I interpret as an invitation to follow her. Boom! Crash! She trips over the floor pillows, but is up again in an instant with no sign of injury. I follow along, noting how alive and alert I must keep my attention to not experience the sting of the fall. This circling, crashing, and up again pattern continues for quite a while, until finally, we both land on the pillows and together roll to a stop.
>
> I look at Mom, whose arms are folded tightly across her tensely held torso as she observes her daughter. "Angie! Slow down!" she shouts, and starts to apologize for Angie's behavior. I laugh gently and smile at Angie, who looks at me from over her shoulder, and then to Mom. I want to assure them both that I am here to learn about their experience and to help. I look at Mom and say playfully, "I see what you mean!" I'm referring to our intake call earlier this week, when Mom shared that Angie was constantly on the go and had some self-control and social issues that were causing difficulties at home and in preschool. Angie, bright and smart, could be sweet and compassionate in one moment, and then suddenly hit you without warning, while laughing. "It is helpful for me to experience how you described Angie," I add with a smile. Then I am off again, following Angie through the room as I "try on" the tempo of her body actions. As Mom nods, a small smile emerges and her body softens.
>
> As difficult as these behaviors can be, what strikes me as I embody Angie's actions is the tempo in which she moves her whole body. A sense of urgency and panic is palpable, evoking a feeling of emergency in me, best described using the musical term *prestissimo*. Defined as "very, very fast, as fast as possible," even faster than *presto* (over 200 beats per minute [bpm]), I wonder what in Angie's past or current life is fueling her pulsing pace. The sense of emergency Angie brings is juxtaposed with the calm, quiet of my studio office and arouses the sensations I feel at the pediatric medical hospital.

I also wonder if Angie has had any prior medical conditions. My suspicions are confirmed the next week in our parent session, when Mom and Dad share that a kidney (reflux) abnormality was detected by a routine ultrasound in the third trimester, requiring a cesarean birth and subsequent admission to the NICU. Though this occurred four years ago, the impact of their experience is still present as their whole demeanor shifts, facial expressions tighten, and their bodies remain still, as if frozen in place. Their despair, anxiety, and fear fill the room as Mom whispers in a stilted voice, "We were so scared . . . . We didn't know what we were doing . . . . We still don't know what we are doing!"

I gently nod my head in time with Mom's statements, and then pause before responding. I want them to know I am deeply listening and feeling their experience. I take a slow, full breath, exhaling before I state, "This was such a difficult time. It was not how you expected the birth of your first baby to go." Hearing this, their bodies melt as their tears flow. I pause again, taking a calm, open, receptive stance. My posture shows I understand, and I am here for the long run. Together we will work through this experience that haunt all their lives. We talk about what aspects of Angie's behavior are most difficult. During this discussion they make the link that her current out-of-control behaviors trigger their memories of feeling helpless when she was born, when their whole life felt out of control.

We discuss the qualities of their felt experience when they are triggered by Angie's out-of-control behavior. I teach them a simple, effective breathing technique, which involves breathing in to the count of three or four, and exhaling two additional counts. We discuss breathing in this way before they approach Angie, so that they feel more in control.

I explain the infant mental health concepts about how young children learn and respond to nonverbal expressions early in life, especially from their primary caregivers. A light seems to go off for them as they nod their heads in understanding and take another calming breath. We discuss how their calmer approach to Angie can help her find and sense her own calmer body. The next week, Dad brings Angie in and says they have implemented these concepts and already seen a difference in Angie and their whole household. Dad reflects further about how his own anxious presence has contributed to the "energy at home."

During our early individual sessions, Angie constructs towers of pillows to crash into and bounce out of. As I witness these actions, I again wonder about her lack of reaction to the strong impact and am drawn to the quickness she employs as she bounces out. Following Angie's lead, I support her to build pillow mounds of varying heights, adding live music to mark her descent, tapping on a tambourine when she crashes and shaking the tambourine to match her quick escape. She asks to play this game each time we have a session.

In parenting sessions, we discuss what the symbolic meaning of these vaulting falls and quick exits might be. Mom and Dad echo each other, stating, "She was so wiggly in the NICU, and we were so afraid she would bump herself we held her so tightly, especially during procedures. She continued to do this at home, and even now we hold her tightly to get her to stop moving. She is so on the run all the time!" We discuss their reactions to her behavior and how it has inadvertently become linked to the hospital experience. Separating their emotional reactions from Angie's needs, they acknowledge the importance of Angie feeling she can move without restraint. We come up with ways to organize Angie's "wild" running sprees around the house by creating a similar game to the one we do in session, when Angie seems to need to let off steam.

The next week, Dad asks if he can come to Angie's session because they have something they want to show me. The excitement is palpable. Dad and Angie construct several pillow mounds in a circuitous path around the room. With Angie taking the lead, Dad follows, crashing and bouncing off the pillows each time Angie exits the pillow space. Their joy is contagious, transforming Angie's behaviors – previously interpreted as out of control – into a dynamic, interactive game.

After a few rounds, I ask if I can add something to their dance-play and they agree. I "challenge" Angie to wait for Dad to land on the pillow mound she is in before she leaves it. With excitement, I jingle the tambourine as she waits for Dad, who gently lands at her side. Angie rolls into him, and they embrace warmly. When he senses Angie's need to "eject" herself, Dad intuitively lets go.

We continue to play variations of this game in the studio with Dad and Mom, and the family at home. Following Angie's lead again, I transition to tapping the tambourine drumhead at a slower pace, as she calmly waits for her parent to cuddle with her on the pillows. As we continue to develop dance-games like this, Angie's parents gratefully report that her wild runs have diminished substantially, and she initiates long hugs without a sense of urgency to be released.

Clinical Discussion

This case illustrates the importance of acknowledging the long-term impact on the parents that may be even stronger than on the child. The parent's experience so early in their parenting can unknowingly and deeply affect their perception of their young child as vulnerable, even as the child gets older and healthier. The now-healthy child can feel the parents' difficulty in letting her explore her environment in healthy rough-and-tumble play, without knowing why this is happening. Helping the parents bring forth their unprocessed feelings about their child's early illness and unconscious concerns about Angie getting hurt enables Angie to experience the proprioceptive and interoceptive input she needs to express her feelings. This improves their relationship and supports a more playful interactive dynamic rather than a restrictive and fearful one.

Conclusion

The main message of this chapter is to be aware of the long-term impact of life-threatening pediatric illnesses early in life – which are associated with pain and invasive medical procedures – on later functioning for parents and children. So, whenever a mental health clinician comes to assess a child's disruptive behaviors and negative emotionality, it is crucial to ask about past traumatic experiences, as parents do not necessarily make the link. The clinical vignette in this chapter illustrates the long-term outcome of a complex interplay of the infant's medical and developmentally compromised condition in the first year of life with environmental factors, including each parent's psychological strengths and vulnerabilities, the marital and parental relationship, and the support system. The psychological treatment with the child started late, specifically at age 4 years, and one may wonder whether her relational and developmental outcomes could have been different if the psychological intervention had started earlier. Different psychotherapeutic approaches may be used. Still, in our experience, the nonverbal DMT approach can open a facilitating window to the parental embodied painful experience, and in that sense, may be more effective than traditional parent–child psychotherapy.

References

Allen, J., Willard, V., Klosky, J. L., Li, C., Srivastava, D., Robison, L. L., Hudson, M. M., & Phipps, S. (2018). Posttraumatic stress-related psychological functioning in adult survivors of childhood cancer. *Journal of Cancer Survivorship, 12*, 216–223.

Anderson, F., & Kunin-Batson, A. (2009). Neurocognitive late effects of chemotherapy in children: The past 10 years of research on brain structure and function. *Pediatric Blood & Cancer, 52*, 159–164.

Annett, R., Patel, S., & Phipps, S. (2015). Monitoring and assessment of neuropsychological outcomes as a standard of care in pediatric oncology. *Pediatric Blood and Cancer, 62*.

Ashford, J., Schoffstall, C., Reddick, W., Leone, C., Laningham, F., et al. (2010). Attention and working memory abilities in children treated for acute lymphoblastic leukemia. *Cancer, 116*, 4638–4645.

Bitsko, M., Cohen, D., Dillon, R., Harvey, J., Kruil, K., & Klosky, J. (2016). Psychosocial late effects in pediatric cancer survivors: A report from the children's oncology group. *Pediatric Blood & Cancer, 63*, 337–343.

Brinkman, T. M., Li, C., Vannatta, K., Marchak, J., Lai, J., et al. (2016). Behavioral, social, and emotional symptom comorbidities and profiles in adolescent survivors of childhood cancer: A report from the childhood cancer survivor study. *Journal of Clinical Oncology*, *34*, 3417–3425.

Carpentier, M., Mullins, L., Wagner, J., Wolfe-Christensen, C., & Chaney, J. (2007). Examination of the cognitive diathesis-stress conceptualization of the hopelessness theory of depression in children with chronic illness: The moderating influence of illness uncertainty. *Children's Health Care, 36*, 181–196.

Caspi, A., Houts, R., Belsky, D., Goldman-Mellor, S., Harrington, H., et al. (2014). The p factor: One general psychopathology factor in the structure of psychiatric disorders? *Clinical Psychological Science: A Journal of the Association for Psychological Science, 2*, 119–137.

Castellino, S., Ullrich, N., Whelen, M., & Lange, B. (2014). Developing interventions for cancer-related cognitive dysfunction in childhood cancer survivors. *Journal of National Cancer Institute, 106*. doi:10.1093/jnci/dju1186

Cheung, Y., & Krull, K. (2015). Neurocognitive outcomes in long term survivors of childhood acute lymphoblastic leukemia treated on contemporary treatment protocols: A systematic review. *Neuroscience & Biobehavioral Reviews, 53*, 108–120.

Fedele, D., Hullmann, S., Chaffin, M., Kenner, C., Fisher, M., Kirk, K., et al. (2013). Impact of a parent-based interdisciplinary intervention for mothers on adjustment in children newly diagnosed with cancer. *Journal of Pediatric Psychology, 38*, 531–540.

Fedele, D., Ryan, J., Ramsey, R., Grant, D., Bonner, M., et al. (2012). Utility of the illnness intrusiveness scale in parents of children diagnosed with juvenile rheumatic diseases. *Rehabilitation Psychology, 57*, 73–80.

Fortier, M., Batista, M., Wahi, A., Kain, A., Strom, S., & Sender, L. S. (2013). Illness uncertainty and quality of life in children with cancer. *Journal of Pediatric Hematology/Oncology, 35*, 366–370.

Gross, J. (2013). Emotion regulation: Taking stock and moving forward. *Emotion, 13*(3), 359–265.

Heim, C., & Binder, E. (2012). Current research trends in early life stress and depression: Review of human studies on sensitive periods, gene-environment interactions, and epigenetics. *Experimental Neurology, 233*, 102–111.

Hobbie, W., Ogle, S., Reilly, M., Ginsberg, J., Rourke, M., et al. (2010). Identifying the educational needs of parents at the completion of their child's cancer therapy. *Journal of Pediatric Oncology Nursing, 27*, 190–195.

Howlader, N., Noone, A., Krapcho, M., Miller, D., Bishop, K., et al. (2016). *SEER cancer statistics review.* N. C. I. Bethesda.

Huang, I., Brinkman, T., Kenzik, K., Gurney, J., Ness, K., et al. (2013). Association between the prevalence of symptoms and health-related quality of life in adult survivors of childhood cancer: A report from the St Jude lifetime cohort study. *Journal of Clinical Oncology, 31*, 4242–4251.

Kohman, R., & Rhodes, J. (2013). Neurogenesis, inflammation and behavior. *Brain, Behavior and Immunity, 27*, 22–32.

Lichtenthal, W., Corner, G., Slivjak, E., Roberts, K., Li, Y., et al. (2017). A pilot randomized controlled trial of cognitive bias modification to reduce fear of breast cancer recurrence. *Cancer, 123*, 1424–1433.

Lieberman, A. (2021, March 8). *Promoting child-parent symbolic play to repair early trauma.* The Spectrum of Play, Online Conference. https://profectum.org/2021-conference-spectrum-play/

Lieberman, A., & Van Horn, P. (2008). *Psychotherapy with infants and young children: Repairing the effects of stress and trauma on early attachment.* The Guilford Press.

Marcoux, S., Laverdiere, C., Alos, N., Andelfinger, G., et al. (2016). The PETALE study: Late adverse effects and biomarkers in childhood acute lymphoblastic leukemia survivors. *Pediatric Blood & Cancer*, 64(6). doi:10.1002/pbc.26361.

Marusak, H., Iadipaolo, A., Harper, F., Elrahal, F., & Taub, J. (2018). Neurodevelopmental consequences of pediatric cancer and its treatment: Applying an early adversity framework to understanding cognitive, behavioral, and emotional outcomes. *Neuropsychology Review*, 28, 123–175.

McDonnell, G., Salley, C., Barnett, M., DeRosa, A., Werk, R., et al. (2017). Anxiety among adolescent survivors of pediatric cancer. *Journal of Adolescent Health*, 61, 409–423.

Oancea, S., Brinkman, T., Ness, K., Krull, K., Smith, W., et al. (2014). Emotional distress among adult survivors of childhood cancer. *Journal of Cancer Survivorship*, 8, 293–303.

Page, M., Fedele, D., Pai, A., Anderson, J., Wolfe-Christensen, C., Ryan, J., & Mullins, L. (2012). The relationship of maternal and child illness uncertainty to child depressive symptomatology: A mediational model. *Journal of Pediatric Psychology*, 37, 97–105.

Price, J., Kassam-Adams, N., Alderfer, M., Christofferson, J., & Kasak, A. (2016). Systematic review: A reevaluation and update of the integrative (trajectory) model of pediatric medical traumatic stress. *Journal of Pediatric Psychology*, 41, 86–97.

Recklitis, C., Diller, L., Li, X., Najita, J., Robinson, L., et al. (2010). Suicide ideation in adult survivors of childhood cancer: A report from the childhood cancer survivor study. *Journal of Clinical Oncology*, 28, 655–661.

Robins, H., Perron, V., Heathcote, L., & Simons, L. (2016). Pain neuroscience education: State of the art and application in pediatrics. *Children's Health Care*, 3, 43.

Seeley, W., Menon, V., Schatzberg, A., Keller, J., Glover, G., et al. (2007). Dissociable intrinsic connectivity networks for salience processive and executive control. *The Journal of Neuroscience*, 27, 2349–2356.

Simons, L., Elman, I., & Borsook, D. (2014). Psychological processing in chronic pain: A neural systems approach. *Neuroscience and Biobehavioral Reviews*, 39, 61–78.

Simons, L., Smith, A., Ibagon, C., Coakley, R., Logan, D., et al. (2015). Pediatric pain screening tool (PPST): Rapid identification of risk in youth with pain complaints. *Pain*, 156, 1511–1518.

Stahlschmidt, L., Zernikow, B., & Wager, J. (2016). Specialized rehabilitation programs for children and adolescents with severe disabling chronic pain: Indications, treatment, and outcomes. *Children*, 3, 33.

Stein, K., Syrjala, K., & Andrykowski, M. (2008). Physical and psychological long term and late effects of cancer. *Cancer*, 112, 2577–2592.

Stewart, J., Lynn, M., & Mishel, M. (2010). Psychometric evaluation of a new instrument to measure uncertainty in children and adolescents with cancer. *Nursing Research*, 59, 119–126.

Stewart, J., & Mishel, M. (2000). Uncertainty in childhood illness: A synthesis of the parent and child literature. *Research and Theory for Nursing Practice*, 14, 299–319.

Stone, A., Broderick, J., Junghaenel, D., Schneider, S., & Schwartz, J. (2016). PROMIS fatigue, pain intensity, pain interference, pain behavior, physical function, depression, anxiety and anger scales demonstrate ecological validity. *Journal of Clinical Epidemiology*, 74, 194–206.

Stone, A., Karlson, C., Heathcote, L., Rosenberg, A., & Palermo, T. (2018). Pain in Survivors of Pediatric Cancer: Applying a prevention framework. *Journal of Pediatric Psychology*, 43, 237–242.

Szulczewski, L., Mullins, L., Bidwell, S., Eddington, A., & ALH, P. (2017). Meta-analysis: Caregiver and youth uncertainty in pediatric chronic illness. *Journal of Pediatric Psychology*, *42*, 395–421.

Tillery, R., Willard, V., Long, A., & Phipps, S. (2019). Posttraumatic stress in young children with cancer: Risk factors and comparison with peers. *Pediatric Blood Cancer*, *66*.

Trentacosta, C., Harper, F., Albrecht, T., Taub, J., & Phipps, S. P., & Penner, L. A. (2016). Pediatric cancer patients' treatment-related distress and longer-term anxiety: An individual differences perspective. *Journal of Developmental & Behavioral Pediatrics*, *37*, 753–761.

Van Schoors, M., Caes, L., Knoble, N., Goubert, L., Verhofstadt, L., et al. (2017). Systematic review: Associations between family functioning and child adjustment after pediatric cancer diagnosis: A meta-analysis. *Journal of Pediatric Psychology*, *42*, 6–18.

Wright, L. F., Afari, N., & Zautra, A. (2009). The illness uncertainty concept: A review. *Current Pain and Headache Reports*, *13*, 133–138.

Zebrack, B., & Chesler, M. (2002). Quality of life in childhood cancer survivors. *Psycho-Oncology*, *11*, 132–141.

Zeltzer, L., Recklitis, C., Buchbinder, D., Zebrack, B., & Jacqueline, C. (2009). Psychological status in childhood cancer survivors: A report from the childhood cancer survivor study. *Journal of Clinical Oncology*, *27*, 2396–2404.

Chapter 8

DC: 0–5™

A Multiaxial Tool for an Integrated Formulation of Symptoms of Somatic and Psychic Distress in the First Five Years of Life

CJ, age 4, was born with hypoplastic left heart syndrome, a rare, life-threatening illness. She comes to my (Tortora) private practice by way of her parents, due to her frequent tantrums, fear of most adults, and hesitant, limited engagement with her peers. CJ prefers to play alone, generally avoiding interactions. She is demanding with her parents and insists on doing tasks, especially those involving her body, such as bathing, dressing, and toileting – privately and on her own. Her difficulties with fine and gross motor development add extra challenges and frustrations to these tasks. Understandably, these controlling behaviors considerably interfere with the family's daily routines. Simple activities such as getting dressed, leaving the house, eating a meal, enjoying social time, and starting the bedtime routine have become huge hurdles.

CJ was first hospitalized when she was 1 month old, followed by more hospitalizations for many months at a time, including 12 operations – three of them open-heart surgeries – before she was three. Cumulatively, CJ spent six months of that time in the PICU. During these hospitalizations, She was with by her parents day and night, as well as other family members and close friends. All the medical procedures, minimal and complex, were carried out with CJ's significant caregivers in the room. Mom reports that CJ was frequently sitting on her or another family member's lap, and they would assist in restraining CJ as she protested during procedures. Once at home, Mom and Dad became well versed in the arduous administration of the extensive medical tasks required as follow-up care.

As they share these details with me, they subtly shift back in their chairs, their bodies becoming tense and still, their arms wrapped more tightly around themselves. Tears well up in their eyes. Their stress about this period in CJ's life is ever present. The sense of guilt and helplessness they experienced is evident as they discuss their complex feelings about needing to support medical procedures that went against every grain of their parenting instincts to provide emotional safety and protection.

Clinical Discussion

CJ's case, presented here in brief, shows the need for the therapist to help the parents make the link between their past traumatic experiences and the child's current behaviors. They were aware that they all felt traumatized

DOI: 10.4324/9781003134800-9

by these experiences, but they did not know what to do about it or how to help CJ with her feelings. They were in therapy themselves, but didn't know how to address the psychological meaning of CJ's behaviors or the more difficult aspects of the experience of illness, including the fear of death. Parents may make the link between the child's behaviors and past experience, but more often than not, they do not dare discuss it with the child.

In this case, CJ's parents are very open and straightforward about her hospitalizations. They have created many photo books of her experiences there, and even have a playful name for her scars from the operations and her feeding tube. They refer to a dance/movement therapist because they want guidance on how to understand the more traumatic aspects of CJ's experience – aspects they knew were held in her body and behaviors. The treatment includes weekly session with CJ, and biweekly sessions with her parents to address their distress and contain their anxiety to enable them to talk to CJ about these more difficult aspects of her illness experience, as well as to get parenting guidance.

The initial goals are to encourage CJ to become more independent with self-care, and for her parents to see her as less fragile and vulnerable. A particularly significant aspect of the treatment includes navigating the emotional and physiological complexity of two additional medical symptoms CJ developed: constipation and enuresis. The medical origins of these symptoms were first misunderstood as being triggered by psychological issues of control rather than issues that stem from her early medical experience.

Introduction

In this chapter, we show how the use of the DC: 0–5™ framework helps formulate emotional and behavioral symptoms children who have suffered serious medical illness may eventually develop, in interplay with parental and environmental factors. Infant mental health is defined as "the young child's capacity to experience, regulate, and express the whole range of positive and negative emotions, to form close and secure relationships, and to explore the environment and learn" (Zero to Three, 2016). These capacities are developed within caregiving and cultural contexts, laying the groundwork for later social and emotional competence, readiness to enter school, and for better social and academic performance (Zeanah & Zeanah, 2019). Despite increased recognition by the medical community that infants can and do show symptoms of emotional distress and psychic suffering, and that psychopathology may be evident early on (Egger & Angold, 2006; Lyons-Ruth et al., 2017), some practitioners are still reluctant to use the term "infant mental health," and even less so "infant psychiatry." For them, infancy does not easily correlate with maladjustment and disorders, and they prefer to think in terms of infants at risk for later emerging problems rather than describing early deviant behavior as psychopathology.

One commonly held view is that the infant is too young to have symptoms of his own because he is completely dependent on his caregivers, and so, at most, one needs to diagnose the latter, not the infant. Of course, the infant–parent relationship is of paramount importance to the infant's overall mental health. Nevertheless, infants are born with their own biological strengths and weaknesses. For example, infants with an easy temperament have the inherent capacity to elicit support and positive responses from others, in contrast with infants with a difficult temperament (Werner & Smith, 2001). Consider also infants with severe physical illnesses, who elicit extreme emotional reactions from those in their immediate proximity. Another common view is that social-emotional symptoms in infancy will fade out with time. This has been refuted by several prospective longitudinal studies (Briggs-Gowan et al., 2006; Bufferd et al., 2012), and for every type of symptom, we can find data about the long-term outcome and prognosis if it is left untreated.

If one accepts the existence of very early psychopathology, the main challenge is then to distinguish early disorders from the range of normal variations in behavior and transient perturbations in development. For example, temper tantrums are typical in young children, but when the tantrums are prolonged and accompanied by aggression, they stop being normative (Belden et al., 2008; Wakschlag et al., 2012). Similarly, impairing separation anxiety needs to be differentiated from typical and normative separation anxiety in 2-year-old children (Egger, 2009). An additional complication inherent in the very early childhood period is that the manifestations of problems may be different at different times of development. This developmental transformation of symptomatology is described as "heterotypic continuity," meaning the symptoms of the disorder change along the years but the disorder itself continues, and adds to the complexity of assessing psychopathology in the early years of life.

Especially relevant to the topic of this book is the need to find a coherent formulation of the infant's symptoms directly and indirectly linked with his severe medical illness and his constitutional characteristics and relational environment. The ultimate aim of making a diagnostic formulation is to plan a coherent and comprehensive biopsychosocial treatment plan. Too often, severe medical illness is seen as the primary goal of treatment, and the psychological reactions of the child and parents are viewed with secondary consideration, especially when they do not impinge on medical treatment. The tendency to separate the soma and the psyche is still powerful in many medical settings, but it is not enough to simply have a psychologist or a social worker on the team; the child's clinical situation needs to be addressed by the whole team in an integrated somatic and psychological framework.

Diagnosis Does Not Mean Giving Up on Our Psychodynamic Understanding and Therapies

The clinician's daily task is to determine whether a given child, at a given moment, expresses sufficient distress or maladaptive behavior to constitute a disorder that requires intervention. Many clinicians find categorical diagnostic approaches valuable in treating young children; such approaches are more helpful at conceptualizing how clusters of symptoms hang together, possibly indicating a need for intervention, than dimensional scores of various constructs (Zeanah & Lieberman, 2019). Giving a nosological diagnosis is a structured, standard way of clustering symptoms into categories that are thought to have a common psychopathological basis. Still, the infant's symptoms need to be understood in their own context, including the child's and parent's own characteristics and psychodynamic intergenerational and transgenerational processes. We must distinguish between diagnosis, the identification and classification of a specific infant or young child's symptoms into categories, and formulation, the way in which the infant's clinical presentation is understood in the context of her risk and protective factors, in her dyadic and triadic relationships, and in her biology, developmental status, and social network. Ideally, the treatment plan should be based on those risk and protective factors that are modifiable, and the therapeutic approach can be either psychoanalytically oriented, attachment-based, or interactive guidance, based on the parents' strengths and motivation, as well as the nonverbal communication characteristics of the child and the parents.

The DC: 0–5 Multiaxial Approach as the Framework to Formulate Infants' Symptoms

In 2013, I (Keren) was privileged to be asked to become a member of the task force handling the revision of the *Diagnostic Classification of Mental Health and Developmental Disorders of Infancy and Early Childhood, Revised Edition DC 0–3R* (Zero to Three, 2005). For three years, we met twice a year in person and had in-between videoconference meetings. The team composition reflected the multidisciplinary approach inherent in the domain of infant mental health: psychology, psychiatry, nursing, social work, and a mix of researchers and clinicians. The ultimate aim of the task force was to compose a user-friendly, evidence-based manual for clinicians and researchers around the world who work with children under age 5.

The multiaxial structure (as opposed to the DSM V, the fifth edition of the *Diagnostic and Statistical Manual* of the American Psychiatric Association), is a very useful way to encompass the complex interplay between the infant's symptoms and his relational context, as well as his developmental competencies and physical health, all within the broader family and cultural context. Axis I is the clinical disorder axis, which refers to the categorization of the abnormal behaviors and/or emotions manifested by the child that cause significant functional impairment in the child's and/or his caregivers' daily functioning.

The criteria of functional impairment overarches all other diagnostic categories because it is the main parameter to help us distinguish between disorder and variation of normal developmental processes. The central diagnostic categories include distinct disorders apparently based on commonalities in their psychopathological mechanisms, while also having specific criteria. The strict criteria for the diagnosis of parent–child relationship disorder convey that not every emotional or behavioral symptom in the infant is automatically the sign of a relationship disorder. Indeed, the infant's total dependency on his primary caregivers often makes people think incorrectly that any symptom in the infant reflects a primary disorder in this relationship, implicitly blaming parents. Thus, in cases of severe physical illness, it is of primal importance to distinguish between those cases when illness and fear of losing the child obviously impacts the quality of the parent–child relationship, and those when there were signs of dysfunction in the relationship prior to the physical illness.

The major diagnostic criteria for a relationship disorder are the child's manifestation of abnormal behaviors *only* in the context of that specific relationship. If the child exhibits additional abnormal behaviors across contexts, she will be given an additional Axis I diagnosis, as comorbidity is common. For example, a child will be considered to have a relationship-specific disorder within the family context if she manifests abnormal behaviors such as aggression, oppositionality, toilet refusal, eating refusal, sleep problems, self-endangerment, role reversal, or breath-holding spells, together with an additional diagnosis, like overactivity disorder of toddlerhood, if the hyperactive behavior is manifested across several contexts. We also need to be able to describe the strengths and weaknesses of the child's dyadic, triadic, and family relationships, regardless of the presence of a relational disorder, as core components of the final formulation of the young child's biosocioemotional status. This is encompassed using Axis II, a dimensional description of the caregiver–child relationship and the caregiving environment (as will be explained in more detail later in this chapter).

Axis I: Diagnostic Entities

It is beyond the scope of this chapter to go into the details of every disorder, which can be found in the DC: 0–5 manual, but we will mention here the diagnoses that are relevant to children with severe physical illness. For instance, sleep, eating, and crying disorders are clustered together since they are all somatic symptoms of emotional distress. In the past, the term "feeding disorders" was used, but has been replaced by the term "eating disorders" (Keren, 2016, p. 498) in order to differentiate the mealtime feeding interaction between the infant and the caregiver from the infant's independent handling of food (e.g. reaching for food, opening the mouth, and swallowing). Not all eating problems are relational: The very young child's eating problem may be linked with sensory aversions, sensory processing difficulties, difficult temperament, or reactions to traumatic medical procedures. In cases when the dysfunctional eating behavior is present only in the context of a specific relationship, the infant will be given the diagnosis of relationship-specific disorder, with the problematic feeding interaction being one of its symptoms, rather than receiving the diagnosis of eating disorder.

In sum, DC: 0–5 defines three main categories of eating disorders based on the child's observable eating behaviors: overeating disorder, under-eating disorder, and atypical eating disorders. Each of these is described elsewhere, in detail, with illustrative clinical vignettes (Keren, 2019).

Eating, sleep, and crying disorders, as well as parent–child relationship disorders, are especially relevant to infants who are medically compromised, as they often co-occur. It is essential for the treatment plan to distinguish between those cases where the illness is the major cause of impaired eating and/or sleeping, excessive crying, or of a disturbed parent–child relationship, and cases where the illness is "only" exacerbating a previously existing problem. But there will be cases where that distinction is impossible to make, such as when the severe illness has appeared in the first months of life, with almost no premorbid normal period of development and relationships. Again, the treatment plan needs to reflect the integrated understanding of the interplay between the soma and the psyche, and to be held in the minds of the physicians and other health professionals on the team.

Axis II: Describing the Young Child's Relational Context

In infant mental health clinical work, the infant–primary caregiver (not always the parent) relationship is often the main focus of assessment and intervention, even when the symptoms originate within the child. Therefore, it is critical to include this relationship as part of the formulation of every case (Zeanah & Lieberman, 2019). Axis II of DC: 0–5 acknowledges the dimensional nature of the relationship between the infant/toddler and each parent/caregiver, and between all family members. For the first time, the triadic and, more broadly, the caregiving environment has received special attention, thanks to the seminal works of (Favez et al., 2009; Fivaz-Depeursinge & Corboz-Warnery, 1999; Mc Hale & Lindahl, 2011; McHale & Fivaz-Depeursinge, 2010; McHale & Lindahl, 2011). For the sake of clarity and standardization, DC: 0–5 has clearly defined the dimensions of caregiving as follows.

1. Ensuring psychological and physical safety.
2. Providing for basic needs (food, hygiene, clothing, housing, health care).
3. Establishing structure and routines.
4. Providing comfort for distress.
5. Teaching and social stimulation.
6. Socialization and discipline.
7. Play and joyful activities.
8. Adequate reading of the child's emotional needs and signals.

It is also of note that DC: 0–5 does not assume that the relationship quality between a young child and one primary caregiver is related to the relationship quality between a young child and other primary caregivers. There is considerable evidence that young children construct different kinds of relationships with different caregivers. Thus, the only way to determine the relationship quality between a child and each specific caregiver is to assess each one directly.

The stability, predictability, and emotional quality of relationships between the adult caregivers are important predictors of the child's functioning. Young children develop important relationships with their primary caregiver and with other family members, who may share a caregiving role with the child or affect the child's functioning through their influence on the primary caregiver's quality of functioning. Young children are keen observers of how, in their immediate environment, adults relate to one another, and they often learn by imitation, adopting the interpersonal behaviors they observe. The affective tone of the adult interactions and their level of mutual solidarity (co-parenting), in turn, influence the child's affect regulation, trust in relationships, and freedom to explore. The specific dimensions of the family caregiving environment include the following.

1. Problem solving.
2. Conflict resolution.
3. Caregiving role allocation.
4. Caregiving communication:
   a. Instrumental.
   b. Emotional.
5. Emotional investment.
6. Behavioral regulation and coordination.

It is expected that the infant's severe medical disease will impact the level of adaptation of the dyadic, triadic, and family relationship, so it is very important in treatment planning to assess the extent to which the illness has impacted the parent–infant relationship.

Axis III: Health-Related and Medical Conditions

This axis emerged from the understanding that the traditional dichotomy between organic and nonorganic symptoms and disorders is a fundamental mistake that has led pediatricians, psychologists, and psychiatrists to misdiagnose children. Body and mind are in a complex dynamic interplay that needs to be recognized when assessing physical, behavioral, and emotional symptoms. DC: 0–5 contains a comprehensive list of health-related conditions (including invasive, painful procedures) and illnesses that are important to mention in the infant's symptoms formulation. The treatment plan for such complex mixed-medical and psychological conditions requires close collaboration between pediatricians and child psychologists/psychiatrists. Axis III is particularly relevant to the scope of this book because we focus on severely medically compromised infants and young children who are undergoing invasive, painful, and repetitive procedures.

Axis IV: Psychosocial Stressors

Here also, DC: 0–5 offers an extensive list of potential stressors for the very young child. The list may be longer for younger children than for older ones because of their total dependence on caregivers' functioning and health. Sources of stress are identified with their duration and cumulative severity. For example, young children who enter foster placements have often experienced more than one stressor, such as neglect and/or abuse, parental psychiatric illness, separations, and poverty. Stressors are divided into several categories: the infant's primary support group (birth of sibling, absence of father or mother, incarceration of parent, death of a parent, domestic violence, abuse, foster care, medical illness of parent or sibling, divorce, substance abuse of parent, teenage parent), social environment (community violence, unsafe neighborhood, immigration, refugee status), educational stressors, economic stressors, infant's physical health stressors (our target population in this book), and legal challenges (child protective services, custody disputes, crime, parental deportation, incarceration).

Axis V: The Infant's Developmental Competence

Five domains of development across the first five years of life are: emotional, social-relational, language-social communication, cognitive, and movement and physical. Scoring is based on four levels: exceeds expected level, is at expected level, expected level is emerging, and under expected level.

Illustrative Example of Use of the DC: 0–5 Formulation

In the case of CJ, featured at the beginning of this chapter, her present-ing symptoms included those related to the parent–child relationship due to her controlling, demanding, and defiant behaviors at home, and those outside the relational context, exhibited as rigidity, withdrawal, and social anxiety with adults and peers, both of which clearly impaired family relationships and CJ's overall functioning. Her DC: 0–5 formulation is as follows:

> Axis I: Anxiety disorder and parent–child relationship disorder.
> Axis II: Level 3 of dyadic interaction.
> Axis III: Hypoplastic left heart syndrome, status post repeated inva-sive and painful procedures.
> Axis IV: Parental psychological distress.
> Axis V: Restricted social functioning.

This multiaxial, mental, relational, physical and environmental formula-tion reveals the need for psychological intervention for CJ, to provide long-term emotional and developmental support as she grows. Selected DMT sessions with CJ, from age 4–6, are included below.

> From the start, CJ's parents are great communicators. Prior to our first session, Mom and I discuss through email how to introduce me. When she tells CJ my name is "Dr. Suzi" and that "I'm a kind of dance teacher," CJ gets right to the point: "If she's a doctor, does she make people better?" Mom is relieved: "This shows she has a clear set of associations with that word, but they aren't all negative. So I think the doctor part is OK." I suggest that if CJ shows more curiosity, Mom explain further that I am

> > a special kind of doctor that helps children and parents share their feelings about anything and everything that may be on their mind, or even not on their mind. We would do it in fun ways that include creating stories, playing, dancing, listening to her favorite music and talking. She gets to choose!

> This introduction works well, and CJ immediately engages, which is significant given her typical shyness with adults.
> The first theme that surfaces is CJ's difficulty with bowel control, specifically holding in her poop and constipation. Over the course of two sessions, the emotional complexity of this theme and its relation-ship to her medical experience become clear. During the initial body–mind–emotional check-in activity that starts each session, CJ picks

the angry, shy, and sad wooden feeling eggs and rolls them across the floor. We run after them, catch them, and send them off again. CJ transitions this play into pushing 12 egg-shaped yoga balls around the studio. Rolling, bouncing, and scattering everywhere, they also bump into us. As we push and dodge them, I reflect on the emotional associations my embodied experience suggests. Anger and "leave me alone" spontaneously arise, evoking CJ's initial feeling choices. In a playful voice, I intermittently shout: "Get out of here! Don't touch me! Get away from me! Who do you think you are doing this to me? I don't like it!" CJ smiles and laughs, her dance-play becoming more determined as she runs and glides around the room.

There is a clear connection between my interpretive verbalizations and her felt experience. She ends the play by vigorously pushing all the balls into one corner of the room and, matching the quality of my verbalizations and yelling, "You have to stay there!" She walks away holding her body tall with an air of confidence and control.

In our next session, CJ immediately initiates this game. This time she opens the studio door just a crack, and we forcibly push and squeeze each egg, one by one, through the opening into the waiting room, where Mom is sitting. The cathartic symbolism of this dance-play is clear. Again, CJ displays an embodied confidence, and Mom reports the next week that her controlling behaviors around her moving her bowels are gone.

Eight months into treatment, Mom shares:

> This afternoon, CJ was drawing, and I brought up her hospital book, asking if we should make a new one with pictures from when she was 2 and 3. She said, "Yes, but you don't need to print out the photos because I can just draw everything." She gave me a hug and wanted to be snuggled more than in many recent weeks. Very cool! Can tell she's working through big stuff with you right now. So glad.

CJ's response is a clear reflection of our work, as we have just started to create a book of drawings from our dance-play stories about her hospital experiences.

In our next parent session, I share how much CJ is clearly creating an embodied narrative about her medical experiences. After the last session, when Mom brought some of CJ's medical toys for us to use, CJ stated, "But what about the dancing? We have to dance!" to which I replied, "Yes, of course we will dance, and can add the toys to our dance-play!"

CJ's controlling behaviors around toileting resurface as day and nocturnal enuresis. This time I suggest a medical evaluation with a pediatric urologist, sensing that CJ may be suffering from weak core muscular control rather than solely an issue of emotional control. Through an ultrasound we discover that CJ's constipation and weak pelvic floor muscles are the cause. In session, Mom makes a link about how their current parenting, monitoring CJ's use of the toilet with constant reminders, may be contributing to CJ's controlling toileting behaviors. We discuss providing CJ with independence and control over the tasks she needs to do for her condition. CJ gets an app that helps her practice her Kegel-like exercises and a children's watch to remind her to drink water to increase hydration and use the toilet. In session, CJ engages in stories using child-size apparatus, enabling her to climb, swing, and jump all around the room, exercising core-muscle control.

At first, these activities work, but after a few weeks, Mom shares that they are all frustrated again. CJ's accidents – and tantrums – have increased. She is refusing to drink her water or do her exercises. In the next session, CJ makes it clear that she is staying in the waiting room with Mom. Taking Mom's notebook, she draws images, and then covers them up with scribbles, requesting that we figure out what they are. I am struck by the metaphor in her actions and verbalize how confusing and difficult this process is with so many unknowns. Mom agrees and CJ smiles, with a relieved nod. Mom reports things have turned a corner at home. In our sessions, CJ initiates a deeper theme.

Next session, with Mom's notebook in hand, CJ introduces me to Charlotte, her baby doll from home who is "very, very sick," with a "super high temperature and 30 operations in just one week. We must take care of her." The notebook becomes Charlotte's medical record, which we use to report her progress both in our sessions and at home while the doll is under the care of "Dr. CJ." Shortly after, Mom reports that their beloved cat of 15 years has died, and CJ has a

> complicated reaction . . . having seen him super sick. When I told her the vet couldn't save him, she got very rigid [and] started asking immediately about when we could get another pet . . . . When I said "Daddy and I are too sad to talk about that today," she wouldn't let it go, and quickly escalated to screaming "You're *not* sad! No one is sad!"

In our next session, CJ states with gravity, "Charlotte has to go through a very serious operation, so we *must* make a *big* obstacle course!" We create a daring course that includes swinging, climbing, sliding, balancing, and jumping through the air. All activities are difficult for CJ to perform, but she places six plush emotion dolls throughout the course to express the obstacles she must encounter while navigating the journey. Dr. CJ tries out the course, enacting each associated emotion, prior to assisting Charlotte through the course. I narrate the adventure, emphasizing the feelings, following CJ's plan:

"[I] see that surprised face," as CJ/Charlotte swings on the trapeze.

"OK," CJ says, "now she has to try the little slide."

I say with concern, "She is worried . . . . She's not sure if she can make it." As CJ gets Charlotte through the tunnel, I state emphatically, "She did it! She was worried, but she did it! Excellent. What's the next feeling?"

CJ walks over to the next obstacle, pushing a circular mat through a tight hole, and I lament, "She's sad that she's not going to be strong enough."

Assisting Charlotte to complete the task with ease, CJ says with defiance, "*No?* She did it!" I echo her enthusiasm.

Next, the mad feelings: "Now, why was she mad again?" I ask. CJ shifts into a shrieking baby voice and tumbles Charlotte. "Oh, sooo mad," I confirm. "She is so mad that it all happened to her and her body. She just doesn't know what to do with these mad feelings and she doesn't want to show her feelings. That we know for sure!"

"OK!" CJ affirms, as she stands proudly.

"And what feelings did we leave out?" I wonder. "Oh! The happy ones – that she made it and she's having her birthday party . . . ."

"OK," says CJ.

"She made it to 1 year-old!" I exclaim.

"No, we're *not* ready yet," CJ instructs, as she prepares the toy cake, complete with candles, flowers, and plates, already planned at the end of our course. We sing "Happy Birthday" with glee.

I add, "We're so happy you're here with us!"

CJ says, "Are you one?" She nods a delighted yes.

I say, "We're so happy you made it to your first birthday. Thirty operations, and this week you just had one a day." CJ helps Charlotte blow out the candles as I continue, "You are getting better and better. Look at you, blowing out all of those candles!"

The medical notes from Charlotte's notebook this week read:

> Charlotte is afraid to go to doctor appointments. She comes for sessions [at Dr. Suzi's] each week because she is worried she will be back like she was in the beginning – sick again. Dr. CJ told her she doesn't have to worry because she will have a party each session. Also, she is a little afraid of the flu shots, but we told her she only must get one flu shot. Also, check-ups are to keep you healthy, so we want to help you not be worried about them. The party can help her not worry so much. And we know the trapeze and climbing are working for your muscles are now so strong.

In sharing this journey with Mom and Dad, we all agree that it is time to introduce more narratives about the precarious nature of CJ's illness. Together, we discuss details they are comfortable revealing and they attend sessions to join in this stage of our dance-play.

Clinical Discussion

This clinical case illustrates how the use of the DC: 0–5 classification is useful to organize complex cases with physical and emotional symptoms, and to plan for treatment. The DMT approach and traditional play therapy have commonalities, but DMT is a type of play therapy with added emphasis on expressing the unconscious material held on a nonverbal body level through engagement with the whole environment. The large physical setting of the room enables the child to act out the felt experiences that she initially does not have a conscious awareness of. Through dance-play, we find the words to describe, narrate, and interpret CJ's unfolding story, creating a link and understanding between her felt experience and verbal processing. The depth of the emotional transformation that occurs when CJ is given the opportunity to physically process unconsciously held experiences is palpable during our sessions. As they unfold, the embodied nature of the child's symbolic play is obvious, and a parallel process occurs between the child's capacity to play out her story and the parent's ability to reflect on the long-standing impact of their child's early memories of this traumatic medical experience.

The child is the first one to take the step through DMT play, and the parents follow her lead. The organization of the sessions occurs organically through the content that comes up in the child's session, rather than it being predetermined. As our individual and joint sessions unfold, CJ's parents are able to understand more clearly how her presenting behaviors are a manifestation of her early unspoken experiences. This enables them to process with Tortora their own unspoken reactions to the trauma, freeing them to put more developmentally appropriate limits on CJ's behaviors and thereby improving the family dynamics.

Conclusion

Babies with medical illness and their families are in extremely complex situations whereby physical and emotional processes are in a dynamic reciprocal interplay. The treating team cannot be divided by "medical" and "psychosocial," but rather needs to adopt an integrative approach. Medical treatments are based on diagnoses. The multiaxial nature of the diagnostic classification DC: 0–5, which includes emotional and behavioral symptoms (Axis I), relational strengths and weaknesses (Axis II), physical illness and painful procedures (Axis III), psychosocial stresses (Axis IV), and developmental competencies (Axis V), could better be used by the medical team as an integrative working model for treatment planning.

Of course, there are pros and cons to making diagnoses in infancy. Cons that have been commonly raised include stigma, labeling, misdiagnosis, and creating resistance in parents. Our answers to these are that stigma is best fought by providing knowledge, and the child's behaviors already label her, often wrongly, as "bad" or "lazy" or "incompetent." Misdiagnosis may be a real pitfall, as it is sometimes difficult to decide whether a deviant behavior is an early sign of pathology or simply an individual variation in normal development. We therefore encourage periodic revisiting of diagnoses. Parents may be resistant at first to hear us giving a specific diagnosis to their young child, but in our experience, explanation of the benefits is very helpful more often than not. For instance, it can be helpful to explain that DC: 0–5 diagnoses in the first five years of life will not necessarily become diagnoses in ICD-11 (the 11th revision of the International Classification of Diseases) or DSM V at school age, as there is room for improvement and change because of early interventions.

There are also many pros to using the DC: 0–5 classification, because it enables us to use shared language among professionals and families, and to make an integrative treatment plan for the infant and parents. It is of paramount importance to stress that making diagnoses does not preclude psychodynamic-oriented psychotherapies, either dyadic or triadic, and does not necessarily mean giving medication. Finally, making clear formulations of the clinical presentation of the infant/young child is a *sine qua non* requisite for conducting the much-needed research on the longitudinal course of infant psychopathology, especially among those who have survived critical illness, and on the outcomes of various treatment approaches that have developed in the last 30 years.

References

Belden, A., Thomson, N., & Luby, J. (2008). Temper tantrums in healthy versus depressed and disruptive preschoolers: Defining tantrum behaviors associated with clinical problems. *Journal of Pediatrics, 152*, 117–122.

Briggs-Gowan, M., Carter, A., Bosson-Heenan, J., Guyer, A., & Horwitz, S. (2006). Are infant-toddler socio-emotional and behavioral problems transient? *Journal of the American Academy of Child and Adolescent Psychiatry, 45*, 849–858.

Bufferd, S., Dougherty, L., Carlson, G., Rose, S., & Klein, D. (2012). Psychiatric disorders in preschoolers: Continuity from ages 3 to 6. *American Journal of Psychiatry, 169*, 1157–1164.

Egger, H. (2009). Psychiatric assessment of young children. *Child and Adolescent Psychiatric Clinics of North America, 18*, 559–580.

Egger, H., & Angold, A. (2006). Common emotional and behavioral disorders in preschool-children: Presentation, nosology and epidemiology. *Journal of Child Psychology and Psychiatry, 47*, 313–337.

Favez, N., Frascarolo, F., Keren, M., & Fivaz-Depeursinge, E. (2009). *Principles of family therapy in infancy* (3rd ed.). Guilford Press.

Fivaz-Depeursinge, E., & Corboz-Warnery, A. (1999). *The primary triangle: A developmental systems view of mothers, fathers, and infants.* Basic Books.

Keren, M. (2016). Eating and feeding disorders in the first five years of life: Revisiting the DC 0–3R and rationale for the new DC: 0–5 proposed criteria. *Infant Mental Health Journal, 37*, 498–508.

Keren, M. (2019). Eating and feeding disorders in early childhood. In J. C. H. Zeanah (Ed.), *Handbook of infant mental health* (pp. 392–406). Guilford Press.

Lyons-Ruth, K., von Klitzing, K., Tamminen, T., Emde, R., Fitzgerald, H., et al. (2017). The worldwide burden of infant mental and emotional disorder: Report of the task force of the world association for infant mental health. *Infant Mental Health Journal, 38*, 695–705.

Mc Hale, J., & Lindahl, K. (2011). Introduction: What is co-parenting. In J. P. McHale & K. M. Lindahl (Eds.), *Coparenting: A conceptual and clinical examination of family systems* (pp. 211–230). American Psychological Association.

McHale, J., & Fivaz-Depeursinge, E. (2010). Principles of effective co-parenting and its assessment in infancy and early childhood. In S. Tyano, M. Keren, H. Herrman, & J. Cox (Eds.), *Parenthood and mental health: A bridge between infant and adult psychiatry* (pp. 357–371). Wiley-Blackwell.

McHale, J., & Lindahl, K. (2011). *Coparenting: A conceptual and clinical examination of family systems.* American Psychological Association.

Wakschlag, L., Choi, S., Carter, A., Hullsiek, H., Burns, J., McCarthy, K., et al. (2012). Defining the developmental parameters of temper loss in young children: Implications for developmental psychopathology. *Journal of Child Psychiatry and Psychology, 53*, 1099–1108.

Werner, E. E., & Smith, R. S. (2001). *Journeys from childhood to midlife: Risk, resilience, and recovery.* Cornell University Press.

Zeanah, C., & Lieberman, A. (2019). Relationship-specific disorder of early childhood. In J. C. H. Zeanah (Ed.), *Handbook of infant mental health* (pp. 467–479). Guilford Press.

Zeanah, C., & Zeanah, P. (2019). Infant mental health: The clinical science of early experience. In Charles H. Zeanah Jr. (Ed.), *Handbook of infant mental health* (4th ed., pp. 5–24). Guilford Press.

Zero to Three. (2005). *Diagnostic classification of mental health and developmental disorders of infancy and early childhood: DC 0–3R.* Zero To Three Press.

Zero to Three. (2016). *Diagnostic classification of mental health and developmental disorders of infancy and early childhood: DC: 0–5.* Zero To Three Press.

Chapter 9

Nonverbal Assessment of Somatic and Psychic Distress

During the initial intake, Jules tells the medical team that she soothes Adele, her 9-month-old daughter with infant leukemia, with the popular ABBA song "Mamma Mia!" She instructs us that Adele does not like being picked up by anyone else but her, and does not like lullabies or other soothing music. Jules demonstrates Adele's ability to calm by singing along with a recording of "Mamma Mia" with Adele in her arms. Adele is immediately soothed. I observe Jules soothing Adele with this song many times, and I too enjoy the rich and dynamic quality of Jules' voice. I wonder whether is it the song or Mom's beautiful voice that pacifies Adele.

When Jules is speaking to the medical team or needs to leave the room for an extended time, Adele is often left with an iPad or iPhone propped up close to her face with a video recording of this song. When Jules is present but speaking to the medical team, Adele's body is alert and tight, oriented toward Mom, with her gaze vigilantly transfixed on her. I cannot engage her.

One day I enter the room when Jules is out and see Adele crying inconsolably and avoiding eye contact. I restart the "Mamma Mia!" video Jules has left for her, but Adele only gets more agitated, flinging her limbs as she rolls her body from side to side in a tense pace, breathing rapidly, still avoiding eye contact. I take a deep, slow breath to calm my body, pausing outside of Adele's crib. I speak to her softly, pausing intermittently, using a consistent tone: "Hi, Adele, this is Suzi. You know me . . . . I see you are upset . . . . I am wondering if you are missing Mommy . . . . I will help you." Carefully, I approach, waiting for her to see me. I reach into the crib, turning off the iPad, and gently pick up Adele. I sense extreme tension and alertness in her body as she holds herself vertically against my upper torso, seeming to push herself away. I rock her in a small up-and-down rhythm, attuning to the beat of her cry, but slowing the pace of my rocking pulse into half-time. Infinitesimally, her body softens into my shoulder. I slow our rocking rhythm again, putting on a classic lullaby, and transitioning our dance to a side-to-side sway. Adele calms even more, relaxing her body as she curls into my torso, placing her head on my shoulder, gazing up at me with a peaceful expression.

Jules enters the room at this time and is surprised by both Adele in my arms and her response to this music. This experience enables us to have a conversation about the origins of Jules' soothing technique using "Mamma Mia!" and opens up our conversation about ways we can expand Adele's repertoire of multisensory soothing skills and help her become more comfortable with the medical team.

DOI: 10.4324/9781003134800-10

Clinical Discussion

In this case, we see that Jules appropriately reads her baby's cues of distress, but she has a limited repertoire of methods to soothe Adele, relying on one piece of music and electronic devices. As with many parents in this situation, Jules' own distress manifests in her difficulty processing feelings about her child's illness and a lack of confidence in her skills to soothe her baby. Electronic devices take the place of Mother's voice. Through the DMT intervention, however, Tortora helps Mom pay attention to Adele's nonverbal cues, demonstrating that it is Jules' voice and facial expressivity that Adele is responding to rather than the song or the use of the electronic devices. This helps build Jules' confidence in her parenting, which strengthens their relationship.

Introduction

The opening vignette sets the tone for this chapter, which discusses how to use nonverbal cues to best support the needs of a baby with a medical illness. As stated by Clancy and colleagues in their systematic research review of studies with infants and young children with congenital heart disease,

> emotional and behavioral dysregulation can result in difficulties with mental health, learning, and quality of life in the long-term, [so] it is important to extend both research and clinical efforts downward in age to focus on the evaluation of infants and young children and identify those most at risk.
>
> (Clancy et al., 2019, p. 3)

This chapter includes research, information about existing assessment tools, and introduces Tortora's (2010, 2011) observation tool, Dyadic Attachment-Based Nonverbal Communicative Expressions (DANCE), adapted here for children with medical illness.

The information cited here focuses on how early-life stress affects the structure and function of the developing brain and the neuroendocrine stress response system, and how the quality of early maternal care responses affect the infant's development of self-regulation. Applicable elements of evidenced-based research are provided to expand the focus to all significant caregivers, including members of the medical team. We review the known physiological indicators of stress in general, and specifically with young pediatric patients who may be at greater risk for later mental and physical health concerns.

The tools presented here provide the medical team with ways to observe and assess the parent–infant relationship, provide screening tools to target behaviors that best support the team's engagement with the baby and primary caregivers, and empower parents to become keen observers of their child's nonverbal cues. Understanding how the young child's cues provide clues to their medical experience can provide the child with an embodied experience of consistent care based on their unique communication style.

Linking neurophysiological stress regulation to later physical and mental health outcomes – and advocating for the need to monitor, assess, and support early intervention – resonates with the conclusions of the research discussed in Chapter 4, focusing on emotion and behavioral self-regulation. The impact of medical difficulties on young children adds to this necessity. A study of the role of emotion regulation and social functioning related to social competence and externalizing behaviors in 69 children ages 1.5–5 years with cochlear implants compared with 67 natural-hearing children found that children with a cochlear implant had less adequate emotion regulation strategies and were less socially competent (Wiefferink et al., 2012). These children regulated their emotions in ways unconnected to social competence, as opposed to the naturally hearing children who relied on social competence for emotion regulation. Emotion regulation did explain externalizing behaviors better in children with cochlear implants, and better language skills were related to higher social competence in both groups. Better language skills, however, were only related to fewer externalizing behaviors in children with a cochlear implant. This research came to the same conclusion as the systematic review studying the early emotional, behavioral, and social development of infants and young children with congenital heart disease, which states that these children experience greater impairment, demonstrating higher rates of externalizing behavior difficulties, and show symptoms of psychosocial impairment detectable in very early infancy (Clancy et al., 2019).

The Neurophysiology of Infants' Distress

Research that examines how early-life stresses affect biological stress response systems, most predominantly the hypothalamic–pituitary–adrenal (HPA) axis, is particularly relevant to understanding nonverbal behaviors in infants with a medical illness. The HPA axis, a primary stress-mediating system in humans, is frequently measured through salivary cortisol, a principle end-product of HPA, by looking at deviations in typical cortisol reactivity (Laurent et al., 2016; Young et al., 2020). Hyper- or hyporeactivity (also known as blunting the system) during frequent or chronic HPA axis activation is associated with dysregulation. Factors such as individual variability in stress-response threshold, the potential existence of sensitive time periods in the first years of life, and the impact of maternal behaviors on the infant's stress-related behavioral reactions and subsequent adjustments have been extensively studied (Gunnar, 2015; Laurent et al., 2016; Young et al., 2020).

Young and colleagues did a longitudinal study collecting data in a high-risk cohort of 112 children born of mothers living below the poverty line and receiving public health care. Nineteen samples of life-stress scores and salivary cortisol were taken between birth and age 37 years to examine the influence of stressors at particular developmental periods on acute adult stress reactions. Their findings are consistent with growing research on the subject suggesting that "early life is (the) key developmental period during which HPA functioning is calibrated, affecting its functioning across the life span" (Young et al., 2020, p. 11). Additionally, early-life stress uniquely influences HPA functioning, predicting "more blunted cortisol responses at 37 years old, over and above cumulative life stress" and "stress exposure in middle childhood also predicted more blunted cortisol reactivity" (ibid., p. 1).

Longitudinal research examining the emergence of stress-response physiology in infants, age 1–3 years, had similar findings, concluding that the earliest years are a critical timeframe for the development of stress regulation. The research of Laurent and colleagues focuses on what qualities of maternal care predict how neuroendocrine stress regulation evolves and affect psychosocial and physical health (Laurent et al., 2016). Infant psychosocial stress regulation was measured by examining the variability and stability of the HPA axis during the first three years by observing infant cortisol levels during mother/infant interactions in regular play and before and after the same stressful scenario across multiple years. Despite individual differences in stress physiology among infants, this research found that – especially during stress exposure and in early development – infants with mothers who were more sensitive and responsive had better stress regulation. This was noted by lower cortisol and more rapid post-stress recovery compared to infants with intrusive mothers, resulting in the opposite effect.

Some evidence also shows that HPA hyperreactivity, described as "non-recovering" consistently high cortisol, was linked to infant distress. These findings support those of attachment researchers that a caregiver's ability to appropriately read and respond to an infant's distress cues acts as a "crucial organizer of the infant's developing capacity to down-regulate negative arousal and safely engage in novel stimuli" (Laurent et al., 2016, p. 1437). Their research "sheds new light on the early roots of stress regulation as a dynamic, socially guided process that impacts basic biological functioning" and highlights the importance of early intervention to support caregivers to develop skills to support the child's regulatory competence (ibid., p. 1439).

Observing Infant States

As discussed in Chapter 4, Wolff is one of the early infancy researchers to focus on observing infant behavior, making a distinction between when a behavior is a reflection of emotion and when it is a motor behavioral state. His research focuses on the dynamic interaction and coordination among the infant's individual motor patterns as these behavior states develop into self-organization. He believes that there is value in looking at how "distinct motor patterns are coupled into synergies, thereby stabilizing the motor system and inducing new coordinated patterns" (Wolff, 1987, p. 97). Emotional expressions that create social communications, Wolff asserts, are dependent on two people and are especially noted during wakeful alert states, including eye contact, vocal exchanges, and imitative behaviors. The emphasis on two people for social communications with emotional content leads us to a discussion about the Newborn Behavioral Observations (NBO) system and its predecessor, the Brazelton Neonatal Behavioral Assessment Scale (NBAS).

The NBAS was developed by T. Berry Brazelton, a prominent U.S. pediatrician and author who was instrumental in supporting the more child-centered child-rearing movement started in the 1950s, urging parents to attune to their babies, especially during specific sensitive periods he called "touchpoints" (Brazelton, 1992). His practices were influential in bringing global awareness to the reality that infants do feel pain and parents should be allowed to stay with their hospitalized babies, a practice that was widely restricted prior to his work. In use since 1973, the NBAS is designed as a behavioral exam to support parents to learn how to track their newborn's changing states of consciousness, including liability and direction, over the first 30 days of life (Brazelton & Cramer, 1990). The exam demonstrates how the infant is able to control and engage in the environment through the use of state changes, revealing his aptitude for self-regulation.

Integral to the NBAS is the caregivers' ability to recognize the newborn's state. Similar to Wolff's behavioral states, Brazelton outlines six states of consciousness in newborns (Brazelton & Cramer, 1990): deep sleep, active (light) sleep, drowsiness, awake alert, alert but fussy, and crying. Understanding a newborn's unique nonverbal ways of demonstrating these states provides clues to the infant's availability to attend and engage. Brazelton was one of the early infancy researchers who saw state as a basic regulatory system. The state the newborn is in will determine the capacity of external input she can take in and use, as well as the type and degree of response the baby will have to environmental stimuli. The ability to recognize a baby's unique ways of demonstrating their current state creates a sense of predictability and responsiveness during an early stage of development that can feel unpredictable.

The DANCE section of this chapter discusses how Tortora expands these six states of consciousness, going beyond the newborn period to read the preverbal pediatric patient's nonverbal cues more accurately. This expansion facilitates a more predictable assessment of the baby's responses and experience, and the caregiver's ability to provide comfort and ease during medical procedures.

The NBO was developed from the NBAS (Barlow et al., 2018). Consisting of 18 neurobehavioral items, the NBO is a clinical observation tool designed to look at self-regulation starting at birth. It demonstrates each baby's budding individuality and personhood, exhibited in the his ability to explore the world and engage in relationships through visual, auditory, and perceptual skills (Barlow et al., 2018). NBO is used in a variety of settings, including hospitals, clinics, and at-home visits, by pediatricians, nurses, doctors, psychologists, midwives, physical and occupational therapists, child-life specialists, doulas, and other infant mental health and early intervention specialists. NBO is focused on the crucial role that attuned parenting plays in assisting infants with their emerging adaptive stress response systems and regulatory competence. Behavioral regulation and physiological states are observed in the NBO to describe how the infant adapts to and navigates internal and external input to maintain homeostasis and achieve self-regulation within the social engagement and building the attachment relationship. By helping parents understand their newborn's nonverbal language, the NBO is designed to promote the caregiver–infant relationship (Barlow et al., 2018; Nugent, 2015).

Like the NBAS, the NBO was developed from the perspective that the quality of early relationships shape brain development and functional outcomes for the infant, emphasizing the important role parents play in supporting the infant to achieve skills in self-regulation, such as crying and being consoled; adaptation to stressors related to the infant's stimulation threshold; and social interaction related to levels of alertness and reaction to human and nonhuman stimuli. The NBO is especially relevant for our focus because these factors all present greater challenges in a medical environment.

The acronym AMOR represents the four hierarchical self-regulatory tasks each infant must accomplish in the first two to three months of life observed in the NBO (Nugent, 2015):

Autonomic/physiological stability includes the breathing stabilization, a reduction in the number of startles and tremors, maintaining temperature control, and being able to receive touch;

Motor regulation is observable in developing control over random movements and a reduction of excessive motor activity, developing good muscle tone and control, and acquiring feeding skills;

Organization of state relates to how the infant copes with stress and develops predictable sleep/wake states, including the infant's ability to screen out noise and other negative stimuli while sleeping, known as sleep protection;

Responsiveness, the fourth task, addresses social behavior, referring to the infant's ability to regulate her attention by sustaining prolonged alert focus toward visual and auditory stimuli and seeking and engaging in caregiver social interactions.

Though they reference the first few months of life, these regulatory skills can be challenging again for a baby with a complex medical condition later in their babyhood and toddlerhood. The Alarm Distress Baby Scale (ADBS), discussed in a subsequent section of this chapter, is a scale used to detect the level of the baby's distress in the first year of life.

Sustained Infant Withdrawal

The concept of relational withdrawal, defined as a turn inward to retract oneself as if to defend and preserve one's integrity, was introduced by Spitz (1946) in his description of anaclitic depression among orphaned infants, and later by Robertson and Bowlby (1952), who described the protest/despair/withdrawal/detachment reactions infants have to prolonged separation from their primary caregivers (Bowlby, 1973). Transitory relational withdrawal is an essential and normative mechanism for regulating interactions in early childhood (Brazelton et al., 1974). When faced with unusual, inadequate, or unpleasant stimuli and interactions, babies show their distress by modulating their relational engagement. Thus, they avoid eye contact, frown, and divert attention away from people and toys, as well as some self-regulatory and soothing activities, communicating relational and/or physical discomfort.

More clinically worrisome is the prolonged relational withdrawal that can be observed in the context of somatic illness, neurological and sensory processing disorders, severe forms of malnutrition, nonorganic failure to thrive, and chronic pain in infancy. Fraiberg (1982) described these reactions as early, biologically based defenses of avoidance, freezing, and fighting. Such behaviors are also frequently observed in children who present with various emotional disorders, including separation anxiety, PTSD, depression, and autism spectrum disorders, and in the context of child neglect (Dollberg et al., 2006). Prolonged relational withdrawal can also be part of a child's response to inadequate interactions pursuant to postpartum depression, especially to the depressed parent's symptom of psychomotor impairment (Puura et al., 2013; Young et al., 2015) and to other parental mental health issues (Mäntymaa et al., 2008). Prolonged relational withdrawal can be considered a mutual adaptation disorder, partly resulting from and always affecting the quality of the child–parent interaction. Over time, chronic relational withdrawal correlates strongly with insecure attachment, infant depression, and language and developmental delays (Guedeney, 1997; Guedeney et al., 2008, 2014).

Measurement of Sustained Social Withdrawal: The ADBS Scale

The Alarm Distress Baby Scale (ADBS) was developed by Guedeney and Fermanian (2001) and is used in several international studies. It is intended for use by pediatricians in routine checkups and does not necessitate intensive training. The clinician needs only to actively interact with the infant by talking, smiling, and touching. The infant needs to be well fed, clean, and rested, and the age range used in the validity study was from 2 months to 2 years old. The scale consists of the following eight items.

1. Facial expressiveness.
2. Eye contact (difficult to achieve and maintain).
3. General level of activity (head, torso, and limbs).
4. Self-stimulating gestures.
5. Vocalizations (pleasure, pain, displeasure).
6. Response to stimulation (sluggish response to pleasant or unpleasant stimulation).
7. Relationship (ability to engage and sustain relationships with other than caregiver).
8. Attraction (the effort needed by the examiner to keep in touch with infant).

Each item is rated from 0 (no unusual behavior) to 4 (severe unusual behavior). The cutoff score of 5 was found to be optimal for screening purposes (sensitivity 0.82, specificity 0.78). It is important to note that the ADBS is not meant to be a diagnostic tool, but a screening tool for targeting a behavior signal alarm that needs to be confirmed, interpreted, and further investigated. To our best knowledge, sustained infant social withdrawal has not been specifically studied among infants with severe, life-threatening illness in the short or long term, other than the scale that was developed in France to assess pain in young children with cancer (Gauvain-Piquard, 1999).

Dyadic, Attachment-Based, Nonverbal, Communicative Expressions (DANCE)

Tortora created the nonverbal analysis tool Dyadic, Attachment-Based, Nonverbal, Communicative Expressions (DANCE) to assist the practitioner in systematically organizing and qualifying nonverbal dynamics of the baby's interactions with her surroundings (Tortora, 2010, 2011). The information gleaned is used to create activities to best support the attachment relationship, and in the context of working with a child who has a medical illness, to provide consistent, sensitive care that is responsive to the baby's nonverbal expressions. Nonverbal observations from other assessment and screening tools – such as the NBO, NBAS, and ADBS – are recorded on the DANCE form to create a comprehensive understanding of individual nonverbal style and the dynamics of the dyad. DANCE provides additional qualitative nonverbal interactive measures to assist caregivers and professionals in assessing the child's efforts for self-regulation in support of both self- and co-regulation within the context of building a strong relationship.

There is a threefold differentiation between DANCE and other assessments and screenings. First, the emphasis on nonverbal experience, revealed through nonverbal cues, exists as its own communicative function. The nonverbal dynamics of the exchange are considered the primary communication, engagement, and intervention strategy. Second is the attention to the subtle qualitative aspects of nonverbal expression in attuned moments between caregiver and baby to glean information about the mover's implicit and intersubjective experience and the nonverbal qualities that make up relationship style (Tortora, 2010, 2013). When working in a medical setting, these qualities are also observed during the practitioners' engagement with the baby, especially during medical procedures. In particular, the qualitative aspects of the baby's nonverbal style provide insight into how he embodies affect states when alone and in dyadic interactions. Specific attention is focused on the qualities the child's actions demonstrate and how he cycles through being calm and attentive, participating actively, getting excited, or overstimulated (Tortora, 2006). Third, the practitioner's self-observations are needed on a body, mind, and emotional level to be aware of how a personal and reactive lens may color their engagement (Tortora, 2013).

DANCE consists of the following ten categories.

1. Body: This category identifies full-body actions and how individual body parts are moved, including postures, alignment, and how the mover balances and shifts weight throughout the body. Noted here are the areas of the body most used gesturally to accompany vocalizations, verbalizations, or when quiet.
2. Facial expressivity and quality of eye gaze: The characteristics and quantity of facial expressions are identified, attending to how and if they support the behaviors of the mover, and how these actions are directed toward the partner. The frequency of eye contact and style of eye gaze between baby and adult are observed, with attention to how and when eye contact occurs; its duration; the intensity of the gaze; whether it appears frozen or transfixed, wanders or is avoidant; and if there is a fluid look and look-away style to match or complement interaction with the adult.

    Tortora finds this category to be especially revealing with the youngest pediatric patients. Even when the baby's actions are limited due to their developmental stage or medical condition, tracking the baby's eye contact and gaze style can reveal their level of comfort or fear with an adult. In typical development, babies' emerging sociability is marked by increased eye contact between two to three months old. There is an increase in mutual gaze, social smiles, and social vocalizations during face-to-face interactions. By 3–6 months, the baby demonstrates skill in reciprocal playful back-and-forth exchanges as she becomes more responsive to social bids. (For an outline of these and other key social developmental milestones during the first three years, see Rosenblum et al. [2019, p. 106]). Absence of this type of playful interaction in the baby who appears to refuse eye contact by turning her head away, averting her gaze, darting her eyes around the room, or not resting her focus, particularly when being held, is especially noted.

3. Body shapes: This category complements the first two categories because it focuses on actual shapes the mover creates in his body when engaging with a partner, such as how the mover coordinates different body parts through postures and gestures during interactions. How the baby shapes her body in combination with eye gaze often provides pertinent clues about the child's level of comfort with different caregivers or medical practitioners. For example, a 6-month-old may tense her body in a vertical stance with a lack of eye contact, as if she is holding herself independently, when in the arms of the practitioner. Conversely, she may mold her body around her mother's shoulder, as if she is fitting into her with an independent body shape and is able to gaze at the practitioner from the comfort of her mother's arms, or she may dissolve her own body weight, creating an image of melting into her mother, avoiding her gaze with the practitioner.

4. Interactional space: Observations in this category focus on how each partner uses surrounding space in the room to engage with each other, noting the distance, proximity, and pathways used to connect or disengage from interactions. Tortora (2013, p. 157) created the term "embraced space" to refer to the intimate connection established when two people use their spatial placement to relate deeply and emotionally. When not confined to a specific spatial distance, this connection can exist in close proximity or across a room. How this embraced space connection is nonverbally communicated through body actions and the spatial placement of the body is noted. Specifically related to the child with a medical illness, we look to see where the child and adult most often place themselves in relationship to each other. For example, is the toddler most frequently in the arms of his parent, or is each parent and child on a separate electronic device, seeming to be in a private world, as a way of coping with stress?

5. Quality of movement actions: This category is influenced by the Laban/Bartenieff Movement Analysis system (Bartenieff & Lewis, 1980), noting the tension, fluidity, speed and tempo, strength (strong, light, gentle, limp, heavy) and spatial focus (direct or indirect orientation to the partner) of the mover's actions. Looking at the qualities of the whole body in action rather than just the face can reveal more accurate biobehavioral responses (Fogel, 2009). How these qualities

make up each person's unique nonverbal repertoire and movement signature, and if these individual styles complement or are opposed to the partner's innate style, significantly impact relationship dynamics. Paying close attention to these qualities while engaging with a young pediatric patient can greatly support the developing relationship. This is exemplified in an attuned caregiver's cautious approach, pausing to wait for the baby to slowly turn her head to look at him before engaging; or when the dance therapist, upon entering the room, greets the baby by nodding her head rhythmically in response to the baby tapping his crib's railing with a quick, strong beat.

6. Quality and frequency of touch: The quantity and style of physical contact, both self-touch and interactive physical engagement, are observed. These parameters include observing who initiates and withdraws contact, the duration of contact, the nonverbal attributes of touch, and when and how it occurs. The patterns of taking turns and pausing, and the quality and frequency of touch each member of the dyad engages, is recorded. For example, to be soothed during a medical procedure, one baby may require being firmly held in a parent's arms while being rocked in a specific rhythmic pattern, while another baby may be overwhelmed by such full-body contact, responding better to a firm hand grasp without touching his body or limbs. Noting the nonverbal details in the quality of the adult's touch can be instrumental in improving the caregiver or practitioner's ability to soothe the baby. Making qualitative adjustments to the tension, timing, and strength of physical contact, such as helping parents become aware of when they are holding their breath or holding their baby with excess tension in their arms and torso, rocking the baby with too much vigor, or stroking the baby's skin too lightly, can greatly improve success in soothing the baby.

7. Tempo and phrasing of nonverbal style: Tortora derives this category directly from music and dance nomenclature, referencing the synergistic experience that occurs when dancing harmoniously together. Here, attention is directed to the unique qualities of rhythm and tempo in each person's nonverbal phrasing sequences. The compatibility and individual differences in tempo, rhythm, and phrasing are observed, creating compatible, synchronous, or complementary styles of interaction.

8. Vocal patterns: This category is especially important with the very young preverbal pediatric population, because their vocal utterances provide clues about their level of comfort, discomfort, or pain. Vocalizations/verbalizations include playful babbling, whimpering, or crying; breath flow; and the volume and length of the utterances. The tone and tempo of the vocalizations are observed to determine if the utterances complement, support, or are at odds with the person's overall

nonverbal-movement style. For instance, gestures typically accompany speech to accent or emphasize intention, often out of conscious awareness, and an imbalance in vocal-gestural patterning implies increased stress. As with the phrasing category, the compatibility of vocal and breath patterns between two people is considered to ascertain if give-and-take pausing occurs during the dialogue, vocally and/or through nonverbal exchange.

9. Regulation and co-regulation: The last two categories (with coherence to follow) summarize observations from the first eight categories and include information obtained from the other scales discussed in this chapter. These summaries can reveal, for example, whether the dyadic interactions between caregiver and child – or between the medical professional and the pediatric patient and/or patient–caregiver dyad – are attuned or create a dissonance. In this category, how each person's nonverbal behaviors support self-regulation on social, affective, multisensory, behavioral state, and neurophysiological levels to facilitate interpersonal interaction and regulation are recorded. The AMOR tasks of the NBO are used as guidelines when applicable. Examples include assessing whether the baby is able to sustain a level of arousal to maintain homeostasis and an alert state while engaging, while noting the qualities of nonverbal input that sustain or interfere with engagement and reciprocity during the exchange. Does the interpersonal dialogue create contingent or noncontingent interactions that support co-regulation between the couple? How might the interactive nonverbal experience influence the baby's neurophysiological development and unfolding attachment relationship?

Though DANCE is not a formal neurological assessment tool, using it to identify behavioral states can reveal underlying neurophysiological processes involved in state organization, and that can be helpful in supporting the infant's experience along the medical journey. Wolff's (1987) observations and initial research analysis focuses on early infant healthy development to describe behavior states, along with Brazelton's (Brazelton & Cramer, 1990) findings that states of consciousness were instrumental when creating the DANCE descriptive taxonomy for young pediatric patients, especially when under stress. These states help identify the young child's regulatory and co-regulatory styles.

Wolff emphasizes the distinct ways each infant strives to achieve a regulated state by creating a motoric synergy, which is observable through the unique combination of nonverbal qualities of their actions. He describes the following behavioral states: quiet synchronous, non-REM sleep; irregular REM sleep; alert inactivity; waking activity; and crying. His emphasis on wakefulness, using the taxonomy of alert inactivity, waking activity, and alert activity, includes the analysis of waking states in older infants (Wolff, 1987, p. 54). Further, Wolff defines

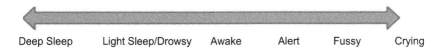

Deep Sleep   Light Sleep/Drowsy   Awake   Alert   Fussy   Crying

Figure 9.1 Arrow Diagram of Six Behavioral States

wakefulness as "when the infant practices and refines acquired senso-rimotor patterns, discovers novelties in the environment, and invents new combinations among component elements that become the means for intellectual exploration and social communication" (ibid.). Motor patterns used to define these states include: vocalizations; facial expressions, such as grimacing and smiling; mouth and tongue actions; hand-face and hand-mouth contacts; sucking hands; respiration; postural tonus; and limb actions, including arm movements and the extension and/or flexion of the knees in kicking. Building upon Wolff, the BNAS, NBO, and other works on state regulation (Zeanah, 2019), DANCE has adopted six behavioral states to reflect how the baby or young child move from sleep to awake to distress along a continuum to acquire self-regulation: Deep sleep; light sleep; awake; three alert states: quiet alert, active alert, vigilant alert; fussy; and crying.

DANCE Behavioral States

Six behavioral states describe the young child's state from sleep to awake to distress along a continuum. Every child has a unique way of transitioning from each state and may not initially move smoothly through these states. Learning to identify related behaviors enables caregivers to support their child in developing more control while transitioning through these states, achieving self-regulation. In each state, it is important to note the posture the baby naturally takes, attending to the position of the head, arms, legs, and torso; eye gaze; and breathing pattern.

1. Deep sleep:

    a. Not easily awakened; noise and light are not disruptive.
    b. Minimal limb movement with only intermittent "jerky," startle-like actions.
    c. Regular and rhythmic breathing.

2. Light sleep/drowsy:

    a. Signs of dreaming, including fluttery eyelids, eyes intermittently opening/closing, an unfocused gaze when open, and eyes may roll back into sockets before closing.

    b. Facial actions, including smiles and grimaces, with additional intermittent mouth/tongue actions without a real pattern.

    c. Breath pattern more variable and irregular than in deep sleep, including brief apneic moments that disrupt the respiration.

    d. Limbs and torso may intermittently move without rhythmic order.

3. Awake:

    a. Face relaxed, eyes open and bright, scans and directs gaze, tracking environment.

    b. Breathing variable but generally constant in rate and fullness.

    c. Limb/torso action readily available, though may maintain more stable posture.

    d. Awake but not yet ready to engage with focused attention.

4. Alert:

    a. The best time to engage, particularly in early infancy, from birth to four months

Three alert substates:

    i. Active alert – obviously engaged/ready to socialize; limbs/body actively moving; audible vocalizing/giggling; joint visual attention.

    ii. Quiet alert – focused attention with limbs/body quiet; eye gaze directed; exudes sense of deep interest, truly taking in environment.

    iii. Vigilant alert – tension/stillness in whole body; appears as if not attending, but actually deeply listening; eyes singularly fixed or darting in frantic manner; some subtle, intermittent perseverative actions; wariness, cautious attitude, with worried, fearful quality; state often observed when picking up tension in room.

5. Fussy:

    a. Appears moodier and more easily disturbed/distressed.

    b. May suddenly fling limbs, kick legs, or throw whole body sporadically.

    b. May throw objects.

    e. Distressed vocalizations.

    f. Can refocus attention, be redirected, or easily distracted, regaining focus composure for limited periods of time.

    g. Can appear tired or near an overtired state.

6. Crying:

   a. Intense vocalizations clearly indicate stress, from whimpering to loud screaming.
   b. Face active, including grimacing, and can be flushed, tears often present.
   c. Behaviors accompanied by diffuse limb/body actions, such as flailing or rigidity.
   d. Breathing patterns contingent to crying pattern.

When applying these states in the medical environment, emphasis is placed on the three alert subcategories to help parents and medical staff members detect the pediatric patient's unique nonverbal cues and best facilitate social engagement. Tortora created vigilant alert from her observations of infants' reactions, especially during medical procedures. Vigilant alert, which occurs under severe stress, can be considered a cousin to relational withdrawal because it has some similar characteristics. The baby's facial expression is fixed, not smiling or frowning. The baby's eye contact, however, appears to be singularly focused on the caregiver, medical professional, or an object rather than withdrawn; or the baby's eyes are darting around in a frantic manner not fixed on anyone or anything. There is an overall stillness and tension to the baby's whole body, juxtaposed at times by subtle, intermittent, perseverative, small, gestural body-part actions. Vigilant alert may be the baby's attempt to modulate relational engagement when severely stressed. The fixed-eye contact can appear similar to the "obligatory attention" of Rothbart et al. (2011), orienting behavior that occurs under age 4 months when the baby cannot disengage his orientation toward distressful stimuli. As discussed in Chapter 3, orienting is a precursor to the infant obtaining self-regulation. Understanding each baby's unique nonverbal qualities in portraying this vigilant state, which occurs beyond 4 months of age, can help the professional support the baby to reorient her attention, experiencing the distress modulated through social co-regulation.

10. Coherence: Wolff (1987) emphasizes using this metric in his discussion about state variables to analyze their developmental change patterns. For Wolff, using coherence as a variable emphasizes the dynamic interactions and synchronies between active concurrent motor patterns that facilitate the self-organization of behavioral states. DANCE also includes a coherence category to highlight the interactive dynamics within the individual and the caregiver–infant dyad that contribute to a trusting felt experience in the relationship

(Tortora, 2013). This includes whether and how a harmonious, co-regulated give-and-take connection is formed and reviewing how the DANCE elements create a co-regulatory experience. Who initiates the emotional and physical connection? How it is communicated nonverbally? Does it create a sense of discord or resonance in the dyadic interaction? This is especially important in creating a sense of trust and safety for a preverbal or pediatric patient with their caregiver and the medical practitioner. Appendix A provides an example of Tortora's process using the DANCE tool for analysis and in the description of her dancing dialogue with Adele in the opening vignette.

A thorough explanation of all of these categories is found elsewhere (Tortora, 2010, 2012, 2013), while here we provided shorter descriptions highlighting the most important categories in working with the young medically ill population and their caregivers.

Conclusion

The opening vignette of this chapter illustrates the clinical use of DMT intervention. The therapist's sensitive attunement to Adele's nonverbal cues demonstrates how young babies regulate differently with different people, and in particular, when the mother is or is not present. Importantly, although Adele was crying, she did not withdraw and was able to reach a co-regulated state with another person. Prior to this DMT intervention, Jules, Adele's mother, did not know that this was possible. Showing Jules that her baby could be soothed by a caring professional attuned to her baby's nonverbal cues opened Jules' and Adele's receptivity to more support. The DMT intervention made this possible.

This chapter provides an overview of the nonverbal cues used in a variety of assessment tools to understand the caregiver-infant relationship and support self and co-regulation. Building skills of caregivers and the medical teams in identifying and responding to each baby's unique nonverbal styles of communication provides a felt experience of continuity of care for the young child and supports the development of skills to cope with the stress of a medically ill baby.

References

Barlow, J., Herath, N. I. N. S., Bartram, T., Bennett, C., & Wei, Y. (2018). The neonateal behavioral assessment scale (NBAS) and the newborn behavioral observations (NBO) system for supporting caregivers and improving outcomes in caregivers and their infants (Review). *Cochrane Database of Systematic Reviews* (3), Article CD011754. https://doi.org/10.1002/14651858.CD011754.pub2. (John Wiley & Sons, Ltd.)

Bartenieff, I., & Lewis, D. (1980). *Body movements: Coping with the environment*. Gordon and Breach Science Publishers.

Bowlby, J. (1973). *Attachment and loss: Vol 2. Separation: Anxiety and anger*. Basic Books.

Brazelton, T. B. (1992). *Touchpoints the essential reference: Your child's emotional and behavioral development, birth to 3: The essential reference for the early years*. Perseus Books.

Brazelton, T. B., & Cramer, B. (1990). *The earliest relationship: Parents, infants, and the drama of early attachment*. Perseus Books.

Brazelton, T. B., Koslowski, B., & Main, M. (1974). Origins of reciprocity. In M. L. L. Rosenblaum (Ed.), *Mother-infant interaction* (pp. 57–70). Wiley.

Clancy, T., Jordan, B., de Weerth, C., & Muscara, F. (2019, September 10). Early emotional, behavioural and social development of infants and young children with congenital heart disease: A systematic review. *Journal of Clinical Psychology in Medical Settings*. https://doi.org/10.1007/s10880-019-09651-1

Dollberg, D., Feldman, R., Keren, M., & Guedeney, A. (2006). Sustained withdrawal behavior in clinic-referred and non-referred infants. *Infant Mental Health Journal*, *27*(3), 292–309.

Fogel, A. (2009). *The psychophysiology of self-awareness: Rediscovering the lost art of body sense*. W. W. Norton.

Fraiberg, S. (1982). Pathological defences in infancy. *Psychoanalytical Quaterly*, *4*, 612–635.

Gauvain-Piquard, A., Rodary, C., Rezvani, A., & Serbouti, S. (1999). The development of the DEGR: A scale to assess pain. *European Journal of Pain*, *3*, 165–176.

Guedeney, A. (1997). From early withdrawal reaction to infant depression: A baby alone does exist. *Infant Ment Health Journal*, *18*, 339–349.

Guedeney, A., & Fermanian, J. (2001). A validity and reliability study of assessment and screening for sustained withdrawal reaction in infancy: The alarm distress baby scale. *Infant Mental Health Journal*, *22*, 559–575.

Guedeney, A., Foulcault, C., Bougen, E., Larroque, B., & Mentré, F. (2008). Screening for risk factors of relational withdrawal behavior in infants 14–18 months. *European Psychiatry*, *23*, 150–155.

Guedeney, A., Pingault, J. B., Antoine Thorr, A., Larroque, B., & The EDEN Mother-Child Cohort Study Group. (2014). Social withdrawal at one year is associated with emotional and behavioural problems at 3 and 5 years: The Eden mother-child cohort study. *European Child and Adolescent Psychiatry*. https://doi.org/10.1007/s00787-013-0513-8

Gunnar, M., Doom, J., & Esposito, E. (2015). Psychoneuroendocrinology of stress: Normative development and individual differences. In M. E. Lamb (Ed.), *Handbook of child psychology and developmental science* (Vol. 3, pp. 1–46). Wiley.

Laurent, H. K., Harold, G. T., Leve, L., Shelton, K. H., & Van Goozen, S. H. (2016, November). Understanding the unfolding of stress regulation in infants. *Development and Psychopathology*, *28*(4pt2), 1431–1440. https://doi.org/10.1017/s0954579416000171

Mäntymaa, M., Puura, K. I. L., Kaukonen, P., Salmelin, R. K., & Tamminen, T. (2008). Infants' social withdrawal and parents' mental health. *Infant Behavior and Development*, *31*, 606–613.

Nugent, J. K. (2015, September). The newborn behavioral observations (NBO) System as a form of intervention and support for new parents. *Zero to Three*, 2–10.

Puura, K., Mäntymaa, M., Leppanen, J., Peltola, M., Salmelin, R., Luoma, I., et al. (2013). Associations between maternal interaction behavior, maternal perception of infant temperament, and infant social withdrawal. *Infant Ment Health Journal*, *34*, 586–593.

Robertson, J., & Bowlby, J. (1952). Responses of young children to separation from their mothers. *Courrier du Centre International de l'Enfance, 2*, 131–142.

Rosenblum, K., Dayton, C., & Muzik, M. (2019). Infant social and emotional development: Emerging competence in a relational context. In C. Zeanah (Ed.), *Handbook of infant mental health* (4th ed.). The Guilford Press.

Rothbart, M. K., Sheese, B. E., Rueda, M. R., & Posner, M. I. (2011). Developing mechanisms of self-regulation in early life. *Emotion Review: Journal of the International Society for Research on Emotion, 3*(2), 207 213. https://doi.org/10.1177/1754073910387943

Spitz, R. A. (1946). Anaclitic depression. *Psychoanalytical Study of the Child, 2*, 313–341.

Tortora, S. (2006). *The dancing dialogue: Using the communicative power of movement with young children*. Paul H. Brookes Publishing Company.

Tortora, S. (2010, March). Ways of seeing: An early childhood integrated therapeutic approach for parents and babies [Article]. *Clinical Social Work Journal, 38*(1), 37–50. https://doi.org/10.1007/s10615-009-0254-9

Tortora, S. (2011). Beyond the face and words: How the body speaks. *Journal of Infant, Child, and Adolescent Psychotherapy: Special Edition: The Primary Prevention Project for Mothers, Infants and Young Children of 9/11/2001, 10*(2–3), 242–254. https://doi.org/10.1080/15289168.2011.600131

Tortora, S. (2012). Beyond the face and words: How the body speaks. In B. Beebe, P. Cohen, K. M. Sossin, & S. Markese (Eds.), *Mothers, infants and young children of September 11, 2001: A primary prevention project*. Routledge.

Tortora, S. (2013). The essential role of the body in the parent-infant relationship: Nonverbal analysis of attachment. In J. F. Bettmann (Ed.), *Attachment-based clinical social work with children and adolescents* (pp. 141–164). Springer.

Wiefferink, C. H., Rieffe, C., Ketelaar, L., & Frijns, J. H. (2012, June). Predicting social functioning in children with a cochlear implant and in normal-hearing children: The role of emotion regulation. *International Journal of Pediatric Otorhinolaryngology, 76*(6), 883–889. https://doi.org/10.1016/j.ijporl.2012.02.065

Wolff, P. (1987). *The development of behavioral states and the expression of emotions in early infancy*. The University of Chicago Press.

Young, E., Doom, J., Farrell, A., Carlson, E., Englund, M., Miller, G., Gunnar, M., Roisman, G., & Simpson, J. (2020). Life stress and cortisol reactivity: An exploratory analysis of the effects of stress exposure across life on HPA-axis functioning. *Development and Psychopathology*, 1–12. https://doi.org/10.1017/S0954579419001779

Young, K. S., Parsons, C. E., Stein, A., & Kringelbach, M. L. (2015). Motion and emotion: Depression reduces psychomotor performance and alters affective movements in caregiving interactions (the Oxford Parent Project, OPP). *Frontiers in Behavioral Neuroscience, 9*, 26–36.

Zeanah, C. (2019). *Handbook of infant mental health* (C. Zeanah, Ed., 4th ed.). The Guildford Press.

Chapter 10

From Lullabies to Dance-Play

The Role of Rhythm, Rocking, Song, and Dance to Soothe and Engage Infants and Young Children with Medical Illness

Carolina, age 9 months, is referred to DMT after her stem-cell transplant because of a lack of eye contact, social and emotional withdrawal, and a listless presentation. Carolina spends most of her day lying on her back, because even though Dad is present, he has been hesitant to play with Carolina due to fears about his daughter's compromised immune condition. The goal of our DMT session is to explore with Dad how he can feel safe to engage Carolina while she is in her crib.

I put on waltzing music to fill the room with a gentle yet mobilizing beat, and we watch to see if it attracts Carolina's attention. When we see her gaze focus, we interpret this as her registering the music. I ask Dad to lean into Carolina's crib and softly call her name. When their eyes meet, Dad smiles widely, and Carolina brightens as she stretches her arms out and pulses her palms open and closed. Next, I encourage Dad to move his head to the tender musical rhythm, staying observant of Carolina's gaze, pausing as her attention ebbs and flows. Once their visual dance becomes consistent, I guide Dad to reach for Carolina's hands and to caress them warmly, pausing to give Carolina a chance to register his presence. I suggest Dad begin to slowly lift his hands, sensing if and when Carolina adds her own movement impulse. Using the undulating melody of the waltz as their guide, Carolina and Dad begin a poignant, gliding hand dance, attuning to Carolina's movement initiations.

This becomes a common play for Dad and Carolina and helps build their relationship, giving Carolina a sense of agency as she explores initiating their dance through reaching, grasping and pulling Dad's hands, stimulating the sequencing and integration of her developmental movement patterns.

Clinical Discussion

The important theme in this vignette is the parent and child's reciprocal withdrawal from each other. Dad's fears and anxiety about Carolina's fragile immune condition caused him to avoid close contact with his daughter. Carolina's symptoms conveyed a depressive reaction based on feeling lonely. Using the undulating ease of the waltzing rhythm creates a calming yet engaging atmosphere that draws Carolina's interest. It provides an

DOI: 10.4324/9781003134800-11

external stimulus, enabling Dad to find a way to be close to and play with Carolina. As Dad experiences Carolina's interest, he reconnects with his child, repairing their emotional distance. The vignettes throughout this chapter demonstrate how music and rhythm are used to create social and emotion engagement for the child, their family, and the medical team.

Introduction

"Babies are born to dance," or so states the findings of an article about a Finnish music research group that studied 120 infants from 5 months to 2 years old (Staff, 2010). Babies have a predisposition to move rhythmically, significantly more so in response to the beat of music and other rhythmically regular sounds vs. speech (Zentner & Eerola, 2010). In addition, infants' positive affect is beneficially related to the degree of rhythmic music coordination. Indeed, the research findings of Mazokopaki and Kugiumutzakis (2009) demonstrate that neonates imitate the expressive rhythmic temporal pattern presented in vocal sounds within their first 45 minutes after birth.

Long before babies have full understanding of the meaning of words, they demonstrate excitement and interest in their mother's engagement with them through singing, dancing, and playing musical games with rhythmic gestures. Love of music and dance is universal, and it is vital for group cohesion to sustain relationships and build cultural learning (Malloch & Trevarthen, 2009). Stern (1985) highlights the natural rhythmic quality of social engagement between mother and infant, demonstrating the infant's temporal capacity to control and direct her actions to socialize with Mom. As discussed in Chapter 1, Malloch and Trevarthen (2009) use the term "communicative musicality" to highlight the co-created rhythmic melodic flow of this loving social play between mother and baby. Karp's (2015) research in the 1980s, observing !Kung San mothers' specific use of body-to-body rhythmic actions to soothe their babies who have a shorter duration of crying compared with babies in Western societies, inspired him to include this technique in his "5 S's" technique for soothing crying babies (Barr et al., 1991).

Throughout time and in all cultures, rocking, swaying, singing, and dancing have been used to soothe and engage babies from the beginning of life. There is a long history of the use of music and rhythm in the field of music therapy with infants born prematurely (Loewy, 2015; Standley, 2003) and all populations during hospitalizations (DiLeo, 1999; Magill, 2006; O'Callaghan, 2008; Robb, 2003). Similar to medical dance/movement therapy, these uses include improving quality of life, providing pain relief, supporting physiological and emotion regulation, relaxation, and emotional expression of the medical experience for the patient and family members.

Building on these methods and research, this chapter highlights the integral role the body plays in rhythmic engagement to support emotional expression, regulation, and social interaction with hospitalized babies and young children. It illustrates how body, movement, and dance-focused activities can be powerful tools to support coping in these very young children, and help the caregiver attune to their baby, thus nurturing the caregiver–child relationship while in the hospital.

Rhythm and Entrainment

This discussion begins with rhythm and the process of entrainment because they are two foundational aspects of music therapy intervention that also have great relevance for dance/movement therapy. The role of rhythm in supporting early socializing experiences is a theme of many researchers and theorists in the field of infant mental health. All definitions of rhythm include a temporal regularity, organization, and patterning that creates a pulse. Rhythm, a foundational organizing feature of music, influencing melody, timbre, and harmony, also organizes language and movement. Unique rhythmic styles reveal details of specific cultural customs. Mazokopaki and Kugiumutzakis (2009, p. 189), two researchers studying the innate musicality of infants and mothers in Crete, state that the word "rhythm" is derived from two Greek words, ρυθμός (rhythm) and ῥέω (to flow). Plato, abstract formalist though he was, connected this meaning of "flowing" to body movements and he defined rhythm as "the order in movement" (Fraisse, 1982).

Babies' first experiences with rhythm occur in utero, through their mother's heartbeat, arterial and venous blood flow, and voice; and sucking is the first organizing rhythm a baby performs. The baby's fetal memory enables the infant to recognize rhythm. Long before babies have a full understanding of the meaning of words, they demonstrate excitement and interest in musical prosody of parentese, the culturally universal manner of speaking to babies in lullaby-like ways, characterized by melodious sounds, extended vowels, repeated pitch contours, and a slight pitch range rising to stimulate and falling to pacify (Trehub et al., 1993). Babies attempt to join in their caregivers' expressions, coordinating vocalizations, emotions, and kinetic energy to their caregiver's engagement, which often includes singing, dancing, and rhythmic gestures (Mazokopaki & Kugiumutzakis, 2009). Trevarthen (1980) states that during the first six weeks of life, reciprocal rhythmic movements and imitative sounds between mother and baby create a shared body state, emotional regulation, and a joint social consciousness, which are foundational for intersubjectivity.

Mazokopaki and Kugiumuzakis' research specifically focuses on how infants ages 2–10 months old communicate emotions and feelings through the rhythmic modulation of their voice, facial expressions, and body movements; as well as how "rhythmic narratives" develop in the mother–infant dialogue as mother sings to her baby. Their findings show a natural intuitive musicality in infancy and an inner impulse to dance and coordinate body, vocal, and facial actions with emotional expressivity. These graceful, gentle, complex, or vigorous repetitive rhythmic and polyrhythmic/multimodal actions serve emotional and social communicative functions. Significantly, and important to the focus of this book, they found that music generated more rhythmic full-body dance moves, creating what Trevarthen defines as "synrhythmic" movements of the body (Mazokopaki & Kugiumutakis, 2009, p. 199). Further, Trevarthen states that synrhythmic regulation engages the infants' inborn motives to connect to the psychological state of others (intersubjectivity) and supports mutual co-regulation of the dyad. In conclusion, they stated, the increase in expressions of surprise, pleasure, excitement, and joy when responding to music shows that joyful baby music appears to motivate self-organization and self-experiencing actions of the whole body, stimulating social interactive participation rather than passive listening. The increased emotional expressivity observed in the infants' rhythmic actions, with and without music, links emotional regulation to rhythmic movement expression starting in infancy. Simply put, adding rhythmic movement stimulates and increases expression and regulation of feelings and social engagement.

Condon and Sanders (1974) were the first to recognize that neonate movements are synchronized by the musical beat of their mother's voice (Trevarthen & Malloch, 2002). This level of coordination between mother and baby naturally directs the conversation to the universal phenomenon of entrainment, defined as "synchronization and control of a physiological rhythm by an external stimulus" (Loewy, 2015, p. 176). In physics, entrainment is described as the tendency for independently oscillating bodies moving at different frequencies to assume a common movement frequency when in interaction with each other. Entrainment has since become a key component of music therapy to describe the role of auditory musical stimuli in physical rehabilitation and to foster dyadic emotional connections, such as with a caregiver and baby, as previously described.

In the early 1990s, Thaut and his colleagues researched and developed neurological music therapy, linking rhythm and music to cognitive, speech, and language rehabilitation (Thaut et al., 2015). Their focus on auditory/rhythmic entrainment, in which rhythmic auditory stimulation puts the motor system in a ready state for movement, provides a scientific basis for our clinical application of rhythmic music and movement in dance therapy to support regulation in young children. Entrainment stimulates neuromotor systems of the body, creating a link between the brain, musical rhythm, and autonomically controlled visceral body mechanisms such as breathing and the heartbeat (Osborne, 2009).

Clinical Uses of Rhythm and Lullabies

Building upon this physiological role of music and rhythm, a series of music therapy studies in neonate intensive care units (NICUs) involving babies born prematurely use live music entrained to neonate's vital signs, as to improve neonate functioning and reduce anxiety and fear perception in parents (Loewy et al., 2013; Loewy, 2015; Standley, 2003). Though we are not addressing prematurity in this book, aspects of this research inform Tortora's work with full-term infants with medical illness. First Sounds research uses specific features of music, rhythm, breath, and sung lullabies (RBL), with live music entrained to observable vital signs of the infant, to enrich parent–infant bonding and provide support during the transition from the hospital to home (Loewy, 2015). This "songs of kin" intervention, defined as culturally based personalized tunes passed down from generation to generation, or favorite songs with melodies, creates meaningful experiences for the parents and their babies. The use of culturally specific music fosters a sense of containment, familiarity, safety, and resilience. Tortora has found that the instruments used in live music to replicate womb sounds in Loewy's research are also effective in soothing full-term babies.

A mother's heart rhythm is created using a gato box, a two- or four-toned wooden box that contains the tone. A Remo ocean disc, an instrument that encases a copious number of small metal balls that roll with the drum base, is used to make a "whooshing" sound similar to the timbre of the placenta. The infant's breath pattern is followed with this sound, while the gato box, softly tapped by fingers, is entrained to match the infant's heart rate. In addition to these instruments, Tortora has added three other instruments to engage or soothe infants during medical procedures: the rainstick, to match the infant's breath or crying pattern; a particularly gentle xylophone called "The Wing," which creates a very resonant angelic bell-like sound; and jewel-colored egg-shaped shakers the infant is visually drawn to and can grasp to shake themselves.

The RBL training teaches parents to entrain to the moment-to-moment vital rhythms of their infant's breath rate and activity level, using their own breath sounds and songs of kin to adapt to the infant. The conclusion of Loewy's research states that the music therapists' interventions can effectively extend the infant's activity level, support self-regulation, strengthen a positive quiet-alert state and induce sleep, and support the parents' expression of grief and promote hope, creating a sense of security and containment. Though infants born full-term who are then hospitalized due to medical illness may not have the same neurological fragility of a baby with prematurity, their medical conditions can cause regression and/ or heighten sensitivities to external and internal sensations. The following vignette demonstrates how Tortora uses a culturally relevant children's song to nurture the parent–infant relationship and help a 5-month-old cope with her mother's absence.

Amara, age 5 months, has recently come to the hospital from abroad, for treatment of severe combined immunodeficiency (SCID). She spends much of her time with nursing assistants because her mom, Aisha, must attend to her older siblings at their temporary apartment. I have had three dance therapy sessions with Amara using a variety of songs to engage her, including popular lullabies and children's songs most respond to, but I also searched the internet for classic Arabic songs Amara might know. In each session, Amara is initially hesitant, but does eventually appear curious, turning her body and gaze toward me in response to the songs I play, letting me hold her hands while I bounce or sway her to the beat. Her expression remains curious, but not fully relaxed or playful.

On this particular day, I enter the room and it is dark. As I acclimate, I see that Aisha is here and has just finished feeding Amara. Using an interpreter, I introduce myself, and we chat for a few minutes about her and how she feels Amara is doing. She is shy, yet warm and interested in hearing how I have been helping Amara. I share my music and dance activities, and then ask Aisha how she plays with Amara at home. She explains that Amara, surrounded by her older siblings, is frequently exposed to an Arabic animation video about a "mischievous boy" who does playfully devious things. The storyline is told through a playful, syncopated, upbeat Arabic song that Amara really enjoys. I listen to it closely, realizing the song is sung in English but with an Arabic linguistic metric rhythm, which I at first do not identify as English. As the song plays, Amara, who is resting on the cushion of the chair, becomes active and alert, flexing and extending her limbs in approximation to the beat. Mom's broad smile and slight nod to the rhythm reveal her own enjoyment with her daughter.

After taking out two small egg shakers, I hand one to Mom, and we shake to the beat along with Amara. With her eyes on Mom, Amara pulses her limbs with increased vigor, interpreting the musical beat. When the song finishes, I thank Mom, and she nods with a smile. I am taken by the scene, reminded of our cultural diversity and the universality of playful ways of engaging with babies. Clearly, the song features a Middle Eastern storyline, but the silliness is universal.

The next week I enter Amara's room, but Mom is not there. A nurse wearing a very worried look on her face is watching Amara in her crib. Amara is clearly uncomfortable, crying and moving her limbs in an agitated manner. I ask the nurse if I can come over and she says, "Please do." She volunteers that Amara needs to rest after a difficult night. She asks me to play some calming music, perhaps a lullaby.

I put on Brahms' "Lullaby". As the soothing cadence fills the room, the familiar tempo deeply resonates with me, but Amara does not settle, seeming instead to be more restless and agitated. Instinctively, I hold Amara close and rock her to the beat. When I lift her, I notice she is very warm (though she doesn't have a temperature), her skin is molted red, and her hair is matted on her sweaty forehead. I swaddle her in my arms, swaying her side to side to the lullaby.

But after a few minutes, Amara is still unsettled. Given her level of distress, I decide to do something unconventional. "What do we have to lose?" I think. I put on the lively Arabic children's video Mom shared with me last week, and the result is immediate. Amara turns her head, riveted to the sound. She shifts to a quiet-alert state, calming her whole body. She purses her lips and creates a soothing sucking rhythm. I pause, in awe of her response, observing her own layering of sensations. I gently rock to this syncopated beat and notice Amara is becoming heavier in my arms as her arms and torso calm. She is no longer sweating, her skin color returns to its natural tone, and her skin temperature cools.

I begin to rock her with more vigor and obvious syncopation, attuning to her sucking, sensing the rhythmic breathing of her body against my own, and listen to her gentle snores. She is fast asleep. Slowly I unlayer each of the sensations we have built. First, I calm the syncopated emphasis of our rocking until my only movement is my undulating breathing, complementing the pace of her sucking and breathing. Next, I gradually separate her body from mine, almost imperceptibly, sensing our lingering body heat. The next part is tricky, because given the positioning of the bed covers, I must rotate her 180 degrees. Maintaining as much of the horizontality I had when holding her against my body, I successfully rotate, placing her on her bedding without disturbing her sleep. Only her momentary exaggerated sucking hints at her body's instinctive response to the shift. I wrap her more cozily in her blankets as the music still fills the room. Little by little, I lower the volume to silent. I pause to watch her, breath peacefully, and feel my whole body calm. In my "mind's eye," I send her images of warmth and love, wondering what her young mind might be imagining, as well.

The use of lullabies in music therapy with premature babies in the NICU, including live singing and recordings, specifically of the mother's voice (Standley, 2003), has also informed Tortora's work, especially with newborn and young infant pediatric patients because both groups require closely observing and controlling the interaction, looking for signals of the infant in distress. Signals of overstimulation seen in both populations include hiccups, grimacing, clinched or averted eyes, finger splaying, or struggling actions. Standley (2003) states that when these signals are exhibited, a 15-second pause is recommended before resuming activity, one stimulation at a time. More powerful cues of disengagement indicate the need to stop stimulation completely to let the baby rest, such as crying or crying facial expression, whining, fussing, spitting/vomiting, or a hand in a halt position.

Music therapists identify the content of the baby's actions and vocalizations using auditory stimulation to match pitch, observing the duration of the baby's eye contact and noting whether she turns her head toward the stimuli, with the awareness that there may be a delay between the infant's awareness and movement production. Masking is a technique in music therapy that uses sounds and music to interrupt the perception of adverse sounds. Similar to this use of music, Tortora has found that matching the infant's vocalizations and/or actions by adding touch or movement, such as stroking the baby or gently rocking in an attuned rhythmic manner, has a soothing effect, successfully causing adverse sounds to recede. Alerting and engaging parents and infants in the hospital is a large part of the dance therapist's focus.

In addition, infants prefer infant-directed singing (ID), which, has a higher fundamental frequency, slower and more regular tempo, and greater emotional expression over adult-directed (AD) songs (Nakata & Trehub, 2004). ID songs modulate infant arousal and are more effective at preventing and relieving stress even over ID speech. Cirelli and colleagues (2018) states that the role of familiar songs is so strong that infants demonstrate increased social preference toward a person they are not familiar with if that person sings a song taught by their parent. Synchronous movement while singing these songs is used by infants to predict affiliation. In conclusion, they state: "When caregivers hold infants and gently rock them while singing a familiar song, they are conveying complex sensory, social, and affective information. These multimodal, interactive musical experiences are likely to have greater impact on infants than passive exposure to recorded music" (Cirelli et al., 2018, p. 70).

The Role of Physical Engagement and Movement in Interpersonal Synchrony

In dance/movement therapy sessions with young pediatric patients, the embodied and movement aspects of these activities are emphasized to provide comfort, to support bonding with primary caregivers, and to create a secure collaborative relationship with the medical team. This later focus is essential, because babies with medical illnesses often engage with medical professionals for many years. Establishing ongoing trusting relationships and positive experiences in a medical setting are vital for continuing care.

A recent research review focused on the "importance of rhythmic movement and socially relevant melodies" in infant's social cognition states that "moving in time with others, interpersonal synchrony, can direct infants' social preferences and prosocial behavior" (Cirelli et al., 2018, p. 66). Interpersonal synchrony is described as a central social component of musical engagement, attained when the movement of one person is aligned temporally with the actions of another, and appears to inform infants' social expectations. Cirelli provides a comprehensive list of recent research about infants and children's musical interactions, ranging from age 5 months to 4 or 5 years old, in relation to prosocial behavior. For example, 12-month-old infants demonstrate a preference for a teddy bear previously rocked in synchrony with them vs. one rocked out of synchrony; once children can synchronize their actions to the beat, they typically synchronize their actions to others; and 14-month-olds act more prosocially with adults moving more synchronously with them and act more helpfully toward those they moved with in synchrony.

Key to our focus is their emphasis on the role of the infant's active experience through rhythmic movement to promote social engagement, stating that the perception of musical timing and movement is interwoven. Cirelli states that when alert and awake, young infants discern changes in rhythm and tempo and, between age 7–15 months, show neural entrainment to the meter and beat of rhythmic patterns. By 5 months old, infants can move rhythmically and exhibit enjoyment demonstrated by positive affect when their actions align with the auditory input; and by 5–6 months old are able to recognize familiar melodies sung to them for one or two weeks, up to eight months later. By the time they are 1 year old, infants take an active role in musical engagements with their caregivers, demonstrated by their ability to perceive tempo, rhythm, and metric groups in musical sequences. The infant's ability to discriminate and entrain to rhythmic patterns, and preference for interpersonal synchrony, suggests that taking time to nonverbally attune to the infant playfully, including through rhythmic songs and games, can build their trust.

The following vignette, featuring Ejaz and his mom, exemplifies how interpersonal synchrony promotes prosocial behavior in infants in musical and nonmusical interactions.

I enter Ejaz's inpatient hospital room, which is dark, as always. It is still and quiet, except for an occasional beep coming from the IV pole from which a medication is being administered through Ejaz's mediport. The quiet at first appears calming, serene. The room is spotless – and toyless.

Ejaz, age 7 months, is in Mama's arms. He is always in Mama's arms, as Mama reports he will settle no other way. I note that Ejaz does not make eye contact with me, or any of the medical staff that keep entering the room. He holds his body curled close to his mom's chest. Mama also holds him very close. She has a forlorn look on her face and often sighs deeply. There is an intense quality to their embrace. I learn that Mama has already lost a baby with this condition. "Who is holding whom?" I wonder. Is it Mama who cannot let the baby go, or is it the baby vigilantly holding Mama, letting her know he is there with her?

During my next visit, Mama is agitated as a nurse explains why she must draw additional blood from Ejaz, a necessary step to do more extensive testing on his condition. Through an interpreter Mama shouts, "You are killing my baby! He has no more blood to give!" Throughout this lengthy, fraught discussion, Mama intermittently exclaims, with a chanting quality, "Oh . . . I know I deserve this . . . . What have I done God? It is my fault . . . ." The pain and tension in the air is palpable. Mama's wail-like sighs increase as she holds her body tightly, rocking forward and backward with a quick rhythmic pulse, as one does when deep in prayer. Ejaz, in her arms, is taken with her. He appears frozen, staring up at Mama's face. It could almost be a quiet-alert state except for his flat, motionless facial expression, which creates the impression of vigilance and fear.

I take out a small shaker and gently shake it, matching the rhythm of Mama's praying body-rock, bringing the shaker toward and away from the baby's visual field. I softly hum, imperceptibly rocking my body, attuning to Mama's rhythm, turning her actions into an expressive dance. Ejaz shifts his attention, turning to look at the shaker. His expression becomes alert and inquisitive as his body softens. In tune, Mama feels her baby's body shift in her arms, and she pauses, her expression warming as she watches her baby engaging with me. Immediately, Ejaz softens his body even more as he becomes increasingly interactive through our gentle rhythmic musical dance. Mama asks, "What is this instrument? Can I have one? He likes it!" And so our dancing dialogue begins. I leave the shakers with Mama and Ejaz. Through our dancing connection, these basic elements of rocking and music-making become the foundation of how Mama comes out of her fearful state and emotionally, playfully reconnects with Ejaz in subsequent sessions.

Clinical Discussion

This vignette demonstrates the concept of illness attributions discussed in emerging literature about the stigma, conceptualization, and attributions some cultures associate with pediatric cancer (Gray et al., 2014). Illness attributions include, for example, the "why?" question, which involves thinking the child's cancer is due to the parents' sins or a failure in parenting the child (Ow, 2003), and a "wake-up call" to live a better life (Uzark & Jones, 2003). These representations may impact the parents' adherence to treatment and their communication with the medical team. This vignette demonstrates the importance of respecting the distinctive way this parent's interpretation of her religious beliefs informs her behavior, using the subtlety of her prayer-like rocking actions to support the mother-baby relationship.

Specific Use of Dance-Play and Action Songs in Intervention

Research on the cross-modal multisensory interaction between body move-ment and auditory beat encoding finds that movement doesn't need to be self-locomotive for the infant to be able to interpret metric beat and entrain, but there does need to be vestibular and auditory input to facili-tate this rhythmic movement and auditory interaction (Phillips-Silver & Trainor, 2006; Trainor, 2007). Infants' perception of musical rhythm is influenced by body movement. Phillips-Silver and Trainor (2005, p. 1430) conclude that "it has long been known that infants are attracted to music and responsive to its emotional content," and that moving the body is crucial and fundamental for the multisensory effect and shapes what we hear. They state that active movement, including simple gestures of the head stimulating vestibular engagement, is enough to support metrical pattern awareness and process beat entrainment. This research provides further supports for the organizing use of rhythm, facilitated by enabling caregivers to soothe their babies by holding and rocking them prior to, during, or after a painful or scary procedure.

Naturally, the necessity of body movement to support rhythmic entrain-ment and prosocial behavior takes us to the use of dance-play songs (Tortora, 2006), also known as fingerplays (Moyses, 2012) or action songs in the med-ical setting. Trevarthen defines action songs as the combination of "melody, words, and schematized sequences of obligatory bodily actions (such as knee jobbing, hand clapping, finger games, and pantomime) into a narrative sequence that provides scope for an infant to participate in predictable ways in interaction with an adult" (Eckerdal & Merker, 2009, p. 250). Action songs are a primary way of introducing infants into their cultural rituals, as the infant partakes in the structure of the melody, the words, and actions of the song (Eckerdal & Merker, 2009; Loewy, 2015; Standley, 2003).

Eckerdal and Merker emphasize that action songs are not meant to solely entertain a passive infant, but to ultimately recruit their lively participa-tion. They state,

> The action song thus epitomized the broad scope of mimesis deployed in human ritual. It draws on bodily posture and movement, gesture, manual dexterity, song, and verbal ability, and their interactive coor-dination into, at acquisition asymptote, a sophisticated formal chore-ography of mutually attuned behavior.
>
> (p. 252)

A salient attribute of these songs that is especially effective when working with the young pediatric population is that participation can follow the infant's developmental abilities, celebrating their maturing capabilities as they progress. Young patients can engage in these dance-play songs receptively, when their age, developmental level, or medical condition inhibits physical engagement, and actively engage when they become more capable. Eckerdal and Merker outline this progression of engagement, stating that during early infancy, these songs bodily engage the baby through tactile, auditory, and visual stimulation. For example, while singing "The Itsy Bitsy Spider," the caregiver may playfully use her finger to move up the baby's body and tickle her under the chin. The focus during these actions is on the infant's spontaneous expressive responses, including excitement, laughter, and anticipatory reactions during repetitions. Baby's motoric responses and initiatives come over time. In mid-infancy, the baby can face his parent sitting close by or on the parent's knee as the parent guides the baby's hands or arms to pantomime the song, encouraging baby's consent by not resisting the actions. By late infancy, the baby and caregiver face each other without physical contact since the baby is an independent participant. The following vignette demonstrates how Tortora used two popular fingerplay songs, with a focus on the motoric aspects of the songs, providing an embodied experience to support a toddler's emotional, and physical regulation.

> Marie, age 2 years and 10 months, newly diagnosed with childhood leukemia, begins her first hospital stay with her single, teenage mom, MaryAnn. Both are understandably overwhelmed. It quickly becomes clear that Marie also has a speech and communication delay and motor planning issues, which manifest in her extreme frustration and tantrum behaviors when she feels misunderstood or frightened. MaryAnn's solution has been to give in to Marie's requests, or give her an iPad.
>
> The medical environment has heightened Marie's behaviors, and MaryAnn has asked for help. As I enter for our first dance therapy session, MaryAnn and Marie are lying in bed, both using their own electronic devices. Toys are scattered on the bed. Upon seeing me, Marie sits up with a startle, kicking her legs and flailing her arms as she screams in a high pitch. As MaryAnn tries to soothe her, Marie throws her toys at me. Mom reprimands Marie, and I pause near the entrance and calmly say,
>
> > Oh, I understand. You don't know who I am and what I might do to you. I am here to play with you, but it will take time for you to get to know me and trust me. I am wondering if you are feeling scared or angry, or perhaps a bit of both.

As I describe Marie's feelings, she pauses with her arm in mid-air and reaches toward Mom, who grasps her hands and pulls her toward her in a warm embrace. MaryAnn looks up at me with an apologetic expression, and again I assure them both that I am here to help. Perhaps, I ask, we should start with a game Mommy and Marie can do together. I ask Mom if Marie has any favorite action songs and she says, "Row, Row, Row Your Boat." What a perfect choice for this moment, given the strong rhythmic beat and active tugging body actions that match Marie's emotional state so well. As we begin to sing the song, I take out a tambourine to add emphasis to the musical pulse and move my own body back and forth with vigor, accenting the push and pull of their actions.

The tone of the room immediately shifts to one of pleasure and we repeat this song over and over again, upon Marie's request, varying the tempo and the style of the push and pull. Seeing how well Marie has responded to this popular fingerplay song, MaryAnn enthusiastically shares the songs she loved as a child, heightening her engagement with Marie. I share our songs with the rest of the medical team, including the nurses, speech and language therapist, child-life specialist, and music therapist.

We use these action songs to redirect Marie's dysregulated emotional state, and over time, rather than greeting me with anger and fear, she now immediately puts down her iPad and stands up on her bed, jumping in a rhythmic beat, and pointing to the floor, indicating she wants to come down to dance with me. The sequential actions and repetitive lyrics of "The Wheels on the Bus," which are at first difficult for Marie to follow, are now among her favorites. She proudly improves her skill in executing the actions, leading us through each move. To support Marie's language development, the child-life specialist creates a chart of the alphabet. Using the chart as a visual guide, I sing the ABCs in a slow, regular beat, pointing to each letter. Marie shows me she understands when she comes over to the chart, pointing and slowing her pace, coordinating the pointing and her verbalizations of the letters to the rhythm. By the end of her over three-month stay, the tantrum behaviors have disappeared, replaced by Marie's new sense of pride.

Conclusion

As stated by the research in this chapter, music, singing, and rhythmic movements such as bouncing, gentle rocking, and dancing with baby are universally used by caregivers to regulate the baby's attention, transition them to sleep, or stimulate playful engagement. Adding this form of engagement for medical staffers that regularly engage with the infants can have significant positive effects, as well. Rhythm is organizing and essential for communication and connecting to others, and it has a physiological regulating and emotionally soothing effect. These temporal measures enable the infant to control their actions and direct their interest in exploring the world in the moment (Stern, 2004). It is through this organizing embodied experience of rhythm that the infant-caregiver emotional bond develops and nonverbal communication builds. Dancing to the beat is the baby's primary way of connecting to the most important people he loves, and can be an empowering intervention tool for the infant with a medical illness and their caregivers, greatly enhancing the overall atmosphere in the hospital, as well.

References

Barr, R. G., Konner, M., Bakeman, R., & Adamson, L. (1991, July). Crying in!Kung San infants: A test of the cultural specificity hypothesis. *Developmental Medicine & Child Neurology, 33*(7), 601–610. https://doi.org/10.1111/j.1469-8749.1991.tb14930.x

Cirelli, L., Trehub, S., & Trainor, L. (2018). Rhythm and melody as social signals for infants. *Annals of the New York Academy of Sciences, 1423*(The Neurosciences and Music VI), 66–72. https://doi.org/10.1111/nyas.13580

Condon, W., & Sanders, L. (1974). Neonate movement is synchronized with adult speech: International participation and language acquisition. *Science, 5*(2), 213–234.

DiLeo, C. (1999). *Music therapy and medicine: Theoretical and clinical approaches*. American Music Therapy Association.

Eckerdal, P., & Merker, B. (2009). 'Music' and the 'action song' in infant development: An interpretation. In S. Malloch & C. Trevarthen (Eds.), *Communicative musicality: Exploring the basis of human companionship* (p. 2410262). Oxford University Press.

Fraisse, P. (1982). Rhythm and tempo. In D. Deutch (Ed.), *The psychology of music* (pp. 149 180). Academic Press.

Gray, W., Szulczewski, L., Regan, S., Williams, J., & Ahna, P. (2014). Cultural influences in pediatric cancer: From diagnosis to cure/end of life. *Journal of Pediatric Oncology Nursing, 31*, 252–271.

Karp, H. (2015). *The happiest baby on the block: The new way to calm crying and help your newborn baby sleep longer*. Bantam Books.

Loewy, J., Stewart, K., Dassler, A., Telsey, A., & Homel, P. (2013, May). The effects of music therapy on vital signs, feeding, and sleep in premature infants. *Pediatrics, 131*(5), 902–918. https://doi.org/10.1542/peds.2012-1367

Loewy, L. (2015). NICU music therapy: Song of kin as critical lullaby in research and practice. *Annals of the New York Academy of Sciences, 1337*(The Neurosciences and Music V), 178–185. https://doi.org/10.1111/nyas.12648

Magill, L. (2006). Role of music therapy in integrative oncology. *Journal of the Society for Integrative Oncology, 4*(2), 79–81.

Malloch, S., & Trevarthen, C. (2009). *Communicative musicality: Exploring the basis of human companionship*. Oxford University Press.

Mazokopaki, K., & Kugiumutzakis, G. (2009). Infant rhythms: Expressions of musical companionship. In *Communicative musicality: Exploring the basis of human companionship* (pp. 185–208). Oxford University Press.

Moyses, K. (2012). *Fingerplays and songs encourage developmen in young children*. Michigan State University Extension. Retrieved July 20, 2021, from www.canr.msu.edu/news/fingerplays_and_songs_encourage_development_in_young_children

Nakata, T., & Trehub, S. (2004). Infants' responsiveness to maternal speech and singing. *Infant Behavior and Development*, 27, 455–464. https://doi.org/10.1016/j.infbeh.2004.03.002

O'Callaghan, C. (2008, April–May). Lullament: Lullaby and lament therapeutic qualities actualized through music therapy. *American Journal of Hospice and Palliative Medicine*, 25(2), 93–99. https://doi.org/10.1177/1049909107310139

Osborne, N. (2009). Towards a chronobiology of musical rhythm. In S. Malloch & C. Trevarthen (Eds.), *Communicative musicality: Exploring the basis of human companionship* (pp. 545–564). Oxford University Press.

Ow, R. (2003). Burden of care and childhood cancer: Experiences of parents in an Asian context. *Health and Social Work*, 28, 232–240.

Phillips-Silver, J., & Trainor, L. (2005). Feeling the beat: Movement influences infant rhythm perception. *Science*, 308, 1430. https://doi.org/10.1126/science.1110922

Phillips-Silver, J., & Trainor, L. (2006). Hearing what the body feels: Auditory encoding of rhythmic movement. *Cognition*, 105, 533–546.

Robb, S. (2003). *Music therapy in pediatric healthcare: Research and evidenced-based practice*. American Music Therapy Association.

Staff, L. S. (2010). *Babies are born to dance*. Retrieved July 1, 2021 from www.livescience.com/6228-babies-born-dance.html

Standley, J. (2003). *Music therapy with premature infants: Research and developmental interventions*. American Music Therapy Association, Inc.

Stern, D. (1985). *The interpersonal world of the infant*. Basic Books, Inc.

Stern, D. (2004). *The present moment in psychotherapy and everyday life*. W. W. Norton & Company.

Thaut, M. H., McIntosh, G. C., & Hoemberg, V. (2015, February 18). Neurobiological foundations of neurologic music therapy: Rhythmic entrainment and the motor system [review]. *Frontiers in Psychology*, 5(1185). https://doi.org/10.3389/fpsyg.2014.01185

Tortora, S. (2006). *The dancing dialogue: Using the communicative power of movement with young children*. Paul H. Brookes Publishing Company.

Trainor, L. (2007). Do preferred beat rate and entrainment to the beat have a common origin in movement? *Empirical Musicology Review*, 2(1), 17–20.

Trehub, S., Unyk, A., & Trainor, L. (1993). Adults indentify infant-directed music across cultures. *Infant Behavior and Development*, 16(2), 193–211.

Trevarthen, C. (1980). The foundation of intersubjectivity: Development of interpersonal and cooperative understanding in infants. In D. Olsen (Ed.), *The social foundation of language and thought* (pp. 316–342). W. W. Norton & Co.

Trevarthen, C., & Malloch, S. (2002). Musicality and music before three: Human vitality and invention shared with pride. *Zero to Three*, 23(1).

Uzark, K., & Jones, K. (2003). Parenting stress and children with heart disease. *Journal of Pediatric Health Care*, 17, 163–168.

Zentner, M., & Eerola, T. (2010, March 1). Rhythmic engagement with music in infancy. *Proceedings of the National Academy of Sciences of the United States of America*, 107, 5768–5773. https://doi.org/10.1073/pnas.1000121107

Chapter 11

Multisensory Dance/ Movement Psychotherapy Pain Management Approach

As I pass by a room in the hospital, Cheryl, a nurse administering treatment, asks me if I can help. After entering the room, I am immediately struck by the scene: Johanna, approximately 18 months old, is crying and kicking her legs uncontrollably, reaching toward her Mom, who is looking at Cheryl emphatically and pleading, "Can't you do something about this?" Mom is clearly distraught that her child is so upset; Cheryl is doing her best to respond to Mom, while attempting to continue the treatment; and I, in my embodied countertransference, am overcome by a sense of fear and aloneness. I wonder, who is attending to Johanna?

First, I must change the atmosphere in the room, as it is clear that everyone is feeling Johanna's physical and emotional stress, but the palpable anguish is distracting and impeding her care. I put on a slow, melodic waltz with underlying ocean waves and take an audible deep breath – everyone notices. Johanna looks to see where the music is coming from, and Mom and Cheryl begin to slow their breathing, matching mine. Now having Johanna's attention, I add a visual layer to the auditory stimulation, rocking the rainstick up and down, matching the undulating wave sounds. Next, I vocally attune to her cries, pairing them to the waves, and they start to take on a rhythmic organization. Mom, feeling this shift, too, takes her baby into her arms and gently rocks her to this rhythmic beat. The tone in the room is calmer.

As Mom continues to rock Johanna, the baby's cries shift into a regular breath pattern and she drifts into what I have come to describe as a meditative state. As Johanna and Mom snuggle, Cheryl is able to continue the treatment. Cheryl and I soon become a team, using this multisensory process with many families to create a healing atmosphere that supports the patient and their parents during treatments that they experience as stressful.

Clinical Discussion

In Chapter 10, we discussed how rhythm and music can engage the child and parent while they are in distress. In this vignette and this chapter, we focus on a particular technique Tortora has developed to help children and their parents during treatments that the child experiences as difficult, frightening, or painful. Specific to this method is the careful attention and

DOI: 10.4324/9781003134800-12

attunement, moment by moment, to the child's responses to a variety of multisensory inputs that are layered in and out, one by one. The sequential structure of this approach provides a sense of predictability for both the child and caregiver, in an environment that feels overwhelming.

In this vignette, Tortora starts by stimulating auditory awareness using a waltzing rhythm with ocean sounds. Next, she adds a visual and rhythmic stimulus to focus the child's attention. Interoceptive organization is reached as she vocally attunes to the child's cries. Proprioceptive and tactile support is provided as Mom holds Johanna in her arms. Through this combination of multisensory inputs, Johanna reaches a meditative calm state – in essence, a sensory-filled interoceptive organization creating a coping response.

Introduction

Chapter 5 focuses on how babies experience, process, and remember pain, concluding with the statement that although babies are more vulnerable to toxic stress related to these experiences, the positive impact of early pain-related interventions that include supportive caregiver–infant relationships greatly mitigates the pain experience. The vignette which began this chapter – describing the DMT method Tortora created to support patients and their caregivers called Multisensory Dance/Movement Psychotherapy (MSDMT) – incorporates the core principles of infant mental health and DMT exemplified throughout this book (Tortora, 2016, 2019).

MSDMT is defined as "the application of DMT with an added emphasis on the role of the body and multisensory experience to support physiological and psychological coping, specifically related to medical illness" (Tortora, 2019, p. 4). MSDMT uses a systematic layering of multisensory input that encourages the child to both engage and regulate their feelings with the therapist and their caregivers to support coping. Activities include dance/movement, improvisation, play, recorded and live music, touch, breath awareness, symbolic imagery, and mindfulness and meditation to augment pain control (Vincent et al., 2007). It is a noninvasive patient-focused method that often includes the parent and is administered in coordination with the nurse providing the treatment. It can be used alone or to complement pharmacological interventions during medical treatments. In essence, it is an "embodied analgesic" that enables the patient to attune to somato-sensorial sensation to engage, soothe, and redirect their attention, building a competent sense of self (Tortora, 2019, p. 4). This chapter provides details of this method, explaining how these activities can have a buffering presence in creating an embodied coherent narrative of healing and empowerment for the patient and caregiver.

The key principle that Tortora integrates from DMT and infant mental health to develop MSDMT starts with the concept discussed throughout this book that our body is a map holding all of our experiences. Stern's sense of self (Stern, 1985) and Tortora's sense of body (Tortora, 2006), concepts both introduced in Chapter 1, emphasize that children process experiences in their body that influence the development of their sense of self. Especially challenging experiences held in the body over time can be somaticized, surfacing as difficult behaviors, or can become traumatic memories that are held in the felt sense. As stated by Lieberman (2021), a specialist in early trauma treatment, preverbal and presymbolic children can experience medical procedures as an attack on their body. They do not perceive the treatment as an effort to heal. They cannot understand the paradox that healing sometimes hurts and how it needs to happen during the cure. A core goal of MSDMT is to create a caring and trusted environment that enables the child and caregivers to cope with their medical experience, building a sense of strength and resilience, developing an embodied narrative that states, "I can do this . . . . I am not alone . . . . I have caring, loving support all around me." During the treatment, a "toolbox" of activities is developed for the whole family to administer, helping them feel empowered with skills they can use to cope with the medical experience. This creates a sense of partnership and collaboration among the patient, caregivers, and medical team (Lee et al., 2021).

Principles of MSDMT

As will become evident throughout this chapter, the child's felt-body experience along the body–mind–emotional continuum guides the MSDMT session. When assessing the young child's pain response, the nature of the child's experience and the dynamic of the attachment relationship between the parent and child are held in mind, because the caregivers play an important role in providing comfort and safety. Activities support the reciprocal relationship between the child and parent, observable in their nonverbal behaviors; the child's ability to communicate their needs and process their feelings based on developmental age; and assistance to the medical team in administering the treatment.

MSDMT is built on the basic principle that children – regardless of age – always take in information on multisensory levels, and this awareness may be heightened during stressful medical events in nonconscious and unconscious ways. This multisensory input impacts how the child receives, processes, and responds to their immediate experience. This greatly influences how the child stores these embodied experiences, registering them on multiple nonverbal and kinesthetic levels that may be felt but not remembered (Gaensbauer, 1995, 2004). Activities are administered by layering specific sensory experiences through playful engagements, which at first distract the patient, then ultimately support them to reach a meditative state when in heightened arousal or perceiving pain. Throughout the administration of the treatment, multisensory elements of engagement are added and subtracted to adjust to the patient's responses. Starting with the first MSDMT session, the patient, caregiver, dance therapist, and nurses gain an understanding of what specific activities best support the patient and the patient–caregiver relationship. These are incorporated and built on during subsequent sessions, creating a toolbox of coping routines. The confidence the child and parent develop is especially evident in later sessions, when they feel able to administer many MSDMT elements even when the DMT is not present. Parents regularly share how much these activities become part of their child's overall coping style, often reporting that the child is able to employ an MSDMT activity during stressful events in their daily life not related to their specific illness (Tortora, 2019).

During MSDMT sessions, the dance therapist is continually considering how the patient's experiences of her illness and the complexities of the medical procedures may impede or restrict the movement explorations that are paramount to the child's emerging body image. Activities are chosen to create supportive felt experiences in the present moment to build positive images that are sensed, perceived, registered, and held by the brain and mind. Porges' assertion of the reciprocal relationship between physiological experiences and psychological interpretations of safety (Porges & Daniel, 2017) is referenced here. The dance therapist's intention is to create a neuroceptive sense of safety by enveloping the child in playful and soothing felt experiences with his caregivers, the dance therapist, and nurses. These social experiences act as a buffer, shifting defensive stress responses to ones of safety. MSDMT activities enable the child to create inner representations of the experience as interpersonal experiences that provide them with a sense of connection and empowerment. Through such body-to-body dialogues, the young patient can create an embodied, coherent narrative of these medical events that is filled with love and care, rather than focusing on pain.

Caregivers' Role in MSDMT

The young patient's caregivers are the most important people in the room when a child has a distressing medical illness, as it activates the child's attachment system. Some infants will have developed a secure attachment, others an insecure one. As discussed at length in Chapter 5, there are many biopsychosocial factors that influence the subjective perception of pain (Charlton, 2005). The developmental age and temperament of the child greatly influence how the child experiences pain. It can be difficult to detect how babies and young children are experiencing pain because their nonverbal distress signals can be difficult to read.

Parents play a crucial role in how their child will respond to treatments that they are all leery of, at best, and very frightened by, at worst. Taking these factors into consideration, the dance therapist strives to help parents feel they have the ability to ease their child's distress. Building a strong social engagement system (SES), as described by Porges and Daniel (2017), during medical experiences that are perceived as painful or scary starts with providing caregivers with a sense of competence in being able to soothe their child's physical and emotional stress. As exemplified in the vignette which opened this chapter, parents become calmer when they see their child more comfortable, which in turn supports the patient, who often tunes into their parent's anxiousness on a nonverbal level.

In MSDMT, this occurs by building a rapport with the parents to learn about their own pain-related perceptions and experiences and their reactions to their child's behaviors. Providing psychoeducation about pain perception in young children can assuage emotional reactions by building a stronger objective knowledge base. At-home activities parents use to soothe their child, including bedtime rituals and playful routines, can be incorporated into the MSDMT program. Including caregivers in administration of MSDMT activities greatly supports the child's ability to cope with medical experiences, and parents feel more competent in helping their child during subsequent treatments when they incorporate MSDMT activities they have learned.

Supporting the Medical Team

The final principle of MSDMT is to provide support to the medical team. As illustrated in the vignette which opens this chapter, engaging the patient and parents focuses the attention in the room, creating a friendlier and calmer environment during treatment that is more conducive to maintaining a neuroceptive sense of safety, thus fortifying the child's SES. This enables the nurses and other medical staff to concentrate on administering the treatment. It also creates a sense of collaboration as everyone has the same intention: to support the child and family during their medical experience. Table 11.1 provides an outline of the goals of MSDMT, developed from these core principles.

MSDMT Activities and Techniques

At the most basic level, bringing a playful attitude to the room through movement, dance, and play activities transforms the perception of the treatment for the child and adults. Prior to and at the start of treatment, especially, toddlers and young children may enjoy engaging in physical activities that keep them active, rather than anxiously waiting for the treatment to begin. It enables the child to spontaneously process her fearful feelings, as well as any tension that may be felt but not discussed with the adults present. Having parents participate helps the child feel their

Table 11.1 Goals of MSDMT

1. Create a playful and/or peaceful atmosphere that provides a sense of understanding and emotional support for the patient and caregiver.
2. Create activities that support the expression and transformation of worry and fear related to the treatment.
3. Help the patient feel a sense of control over some aspects of the medical experience.
4. Promote coping and pain management strategies to achieve a "meditative" state marked by a more peaceful disposition, redirection of the patient's attention away from treatment, and less focused attention on pain.
5. Help parents and other caregivers during treatment to feel capable of soothing the child and supporting themselves during the treatment.
6. Create a toolbox of rituals during the procedure that can be practiced at nonstressful times to support additional coping during treatments and other stressful events.
7. Create an environment that promotes a sense of collaboration with the medical staff.

support and also redirects the parents' focus, bringing them relief as they see their child enjoying herself in ways that are typical in childhood. For toddlers and older children, these activities can include playing with a beloved plush toy, throwing and catching a ball, dancing to the child's favorite movie soundtracks, or acting out scenarios of characters they identify with. Throughout the play, the dance therapist pays attention to the specific characteristics of the activity and the nature of the movie or superhero characters the child embodies to identify emotional parallels with their present experience. For example, we marvel at how quickly, through practice, the child can use her strength to get a ball into a basketball hoop, directing her attention toward the achievement. As the child shoots a "Spider-Man web," we emphasize their success in lassoing our limbs around our body, binding our arms tightly around our torso. As the child directs their imaginary Harry Potter wand toward us, they experience strength as we enact being pushed back through the room with force. When they sweep their arms in a circle while singing Elsa's signature "Let It Go," we emulate the power in their voice, by twirling around the room, sweeping up scarves to imitate the thunderous wind.

We also embed practical skills within the stories the children embody to practice coping techniques they will use when they experience pain. The child may blow the rainbow scarves up into the air to spread "rainbow magic around the room," exercising breathing skills or blowing bubbles, catching and popping them as they fall with the image of targeting the cancer cells the medicine is destroying. As the child sings, dances, and acts, we use the opportunity to narrate themes that include facing difficult feelings, navigating the unknown, being able to overcome obstacles, and feeling strong. Through the metaphors embedded in these embodied stories and activities, we acknowledge the struggles of the current experience while creating a sense of empowerment. These activities enable the children to express and harness their fears and worries and experience a sense of control within the context of treatment that is in many ways out of their control.

Body–Mind–Emotional Continuum in MSDMT

These examples and the underlying structure and duration of the specific activities in the MSDMT method build upon the body–mind–emotional continuum discussed throughout this book. Activities are based on the principle that there is a circular connection between how these three elements of self influence each other: We enter into a dialogue with the patient by attending to their body experience; what we perceive might be on their mind and their shifting emotional state, observable through their nonverbal behaviors, vocalizations, and verbalizations. The physical activities stimulate their body experience. The use of imagery, guided visualizations, and with older toddlers and children, the use of simple language to hold their attention – such as counting their inhales and exhales, explaining their immediate experience related to medical procedures, like why they are hearing a beeping noise from equipment, or preparing them for a gentle squeeze on their arm when the nurse takes a blood pressure reading – focuses their mind. Their emotions are supported by creating activities and stories that enable them to embody and metaphorically express their feelings and maintain the security of the parent–child relationship.

Finally, as discussed in Chapter 3, using our bodies as an additional tool, the dance therapist also pays keen attention to her own embodied countertransference experience throughout the session. This focus provides information about her personal felt experience and thoughts and emotions that are evoked, which may also relate to the patient and caregiver's potential experience and the overall feeling of the treatment room. This informs her decisions about what to do next.

Layering the Senses

Although the MSDMT session incorporates all aspects of the BME continuum, which elements get emphasized depends on the individual presentation, temperament, and developmental age of the patient. We consider each element as an additional layer of input that is implemented with careful attention paid to the impact it has on the child, caregiver, and the overall environment. The activities are chosen and administered through the DMT techniques of attuning to and mirroring the quality of the patient's nonverbal behaviors. The term "layering the senses" describes how to add and subtract sensory input related to the eight sensory systems, which are made up of the five commonly known senses: visual, auditory, tactile, gustatory (taste), olfactory (smell), and the three movement-related senses: proprioceptive, vestibular, and interoceptive. It may not always be possible to completely isolate individual sensations, but being aware of which sensations you are emphasizing and the ones the child attends to most is very effective in pain management. Paying attention to which and how much sensory engagement is administered is important because children can be in a heightened state of arousal when they are frightened or worried, and some treatments intensify physiological and emotional arousal, stressing the child's neuroceptive sense of safety. Each sensory engagement introduces another layer of input, so without meaning to, we can quickly bombard a baby or young child who may be sensitive. Layering the senses is used to both calm and engage the baby playfully.

Multisensory elements are added and subtracted moment by moment to adjust to the patient's responses throughout treatment. Layering specific sensory experiences to achieve a meditative experience is especially helpful for the patient when in pain or an amplified arousal state. A meditative state is identified when the child's observable behaviors demonstrate a focused state of attention and coping, even if elevated vital signs such as a higher heart rate are present. Examples include a strong concentration on guided imagery, maintaining rhythmic breathing, a shift in body activity to a calmer state or more regulated rocking, and eyes often closed. It is important to note that there is a finely attuned aspect to each layer of sensory input the child is focusing on during this meditative state, with each layer playing an important role in adjusting the perception of pain. A subtle disruption of this layering, by attempting to move or talk to the patient, can disturb this state. Recommencing each layer is necessary to resume the meditation. It is this reaction to disruption that differentiates a meditative state from sleeping; when asleep, the child will remain asleep despite the disruption.

Learning how to identify the sensory actions that best support the young patient also helps caregivers feel confident about being able to soothe their child. The ordering of senses is personal for each child and their caregivers. A description of and specific activities used in each of the eight sensory systems are described in Table 11.2, which provides tips to keep in mind when administering the concept of layering the senses. Examples of a MSDMT session plan with an infant and a toddler are provided in Appendix B.

Interoception

Interoception refers to the moment-to-moment nervous system process that senses, interprets, integrates, and maps signals originating in the body, across unconscious and conscious levels, to maintain a homeostatic

Table 11.2 Tips for Layering Senses – Supporting Parent's Participation

1. Before engaging with your child, attune to your own breath quality.
   a. First, notice the quality of your inhale and exhale without changing it.
   b. After you notice it, breathe in for a count of three or four, and then pause and exhale for at least one or two counts longer to stimulate a more focused body state.
   c. Don't worry about reaching a certain level of calm; any shift toward focused attention and relaxation is effective.
2. Approach, listen, and observe your child from this focused state.
3. How many senses does your child need to stay regulated on a body–mind–emotional level?
   a. Remember, this may change during the treatment.
4. Determine your child's arousal level and notice how each multisensory engagement introduces another layer of input.
   a. Your presence stimulates your child's visual sense, especially when you animate your facial expressions.
   b. Add verbal or vocal utterances to stimulate auditory sensations.
5. Touch adds tactile sensation. The way you touch can add proprioceptive, vestibular, and interoceptive sensations. Pay attention to the rate, intensity, and duration of sensory input to help your child stay organized and in control on a body–mind–emotional level.
6. Add and subtract layers to determine how much sensory input your child can manage.
7. Try these actions while holding or being in contact with your child:
   a. Notice the strength of your hold that best soothes your child.
   b. Notice how you phrase your actions, moving in a smooth and fluid manner or creating an accented beat as you rock or sway your child.
   c. Notice if your child prefers to stay in place, move around the room, or change levels of space from high to low.
   d. When rocking:
      i.   Create an accented regular rhythm.
      ii. Move your child up and down, side to side, forward and backward.
      iii. Notice which direction is most calming for your child.
      iv. Explore varying tempos to find which one is most soothing.
   e. When swaying:
      i.   Create a flowing swing to your actions without a distinct accent.
      ii. Notice how close/far away from your body your child needs to be to be calm.
      iii. Vary the speed of your sway to find which one is most soothing.

balance (Khalsa et al., 2018). It is the system that provides us with the understanding and feeling of what is going on inside our bodies. Body states – including sensations of breathing, tiredness, hunger, headaches, nausea, pain, digestion, temperature, itchiness, and the recognition of our emotion states – are all features of the interoception system. Interoceptive sensing is instrumental in aligning one's embodied self-awareness, actions, and emotional presence in the immediate moment (Fogel, 2009), and is considered the eighth sensory system and a hidden internal sense because it plays an integral role in self-regulation, body states, emotional experiences, and consciousness (Khalsa et al., 2018; Mahler, 2017). Interceptive processes frequently occur outside of consciousness, with interoceptive awareness often coming into play when homeostasis is disrupted. One aspect of interoception that is pertinent to our focus, and is garnering a great deal of research interest, is its key role in how we decide to navigate our surroundings to achieve a state of comfort and ease, as it informs our emotional reactions and state.

Many of the reactive and dysregulated behaviors of young pediatric patients are stimulated by interoceptive sensations that they cannot easily understand or explain. Young patients can become very focused on even the most subtle internal sensations, especially when in a high state of arousal and/or pain. Some medications and treatments have a side effect of heightening pain receptors, amplifying sensitivity to internal sensations, but specific MSDMT activities can help the child regain a regulatory state. Activities that stimulate internal breath awareness can be as simple as breathing in for three counts and out for longer, stimulating a relaxation response. With very young babies, we do this by supporting the caregiver to attend to their own breathing while holding the baby. Attending to the rhythm, depth, and flow of our own breath, especially when the child is in body-to-body contact, acts as a nonverbal guide, soothing the child to relax and synchronize his breath pattern. The physical sensation of our vocalizations, such as sighing deeply on exhale, humming to create a vibrating sensation in our chest, and the breath pattern during verbalizations, are also perceived by the baby. Matching the child's vocalizations, especially if they are crying or moaning, through a method we call attuned toning, helps to direct the child's awareness to other parts of their body that are not experiencing pain.

For toddlers, in addition to counting, we help them become aware of their breath using imagery. Visualizing ocean waves while breathing, for example, engages the mind, providing a visual and felt experience that helps redirect the child's attention away from focusing on the pain. We ride waves up as we inhale deeply, swelling our full chest, and then surfing down with the wave as we exhale. For a gentler ocean image, the child can play on the shoreline, lying on the sand, sensing the undulating tide glide across their body as they inhale, and sweeping back the sea as they exhale.

Tactile System

The tactile system relates to how our body processes information related to touch. Sensory receptors are located in our skin and mouth. Touch can be useful at all stages of treatment, but again, as with each sensory system, keen observation and attention to the patient's preferences is essential.

The way we touch a baby communicates a significant amount of information that we may not initially be aware of. Touch creates a social connection (Denworth, 2015). During medical treatment physical care, touch – from primary caregivers and medical staff especially – plays a significant role in how the infant gets to know his own body in the development of his embodied experience, which in turn influences his developing body scheme. The sense of touch relies on a human's largest sense organ, the skin, and is the first sense to develop in utero (Field, 2014; Tobin, 2011). Unsurprisingly, then, the skin is considered a social organ (Dunbar, 2010; Morrison et al., 2010). Parental touch, and skin-to-skin care in humans, has organizing effects on the baby's stress system (Feldman, 2011; Field, 2014). From the moment children are born, parents communicate with them through touch. To study the role of touch as a communicative signal in parent–infant dyads in relation to neural and physiological synchrony, Nguyen and colleagues (2021) measured the brain activity and respiratory sinus arrhythmia of 69 4–6-month-old infants and mother dyads. Their findings revealed that the highest physiological synchrony occurs during face-to-face interactions, and affectionate maternal touch in face-to-face interactions was related positively to neural synchrony but not to physiological synchrony. Their conclusions suggest that touch mediates mutual attunement of brain activity, proposing that neural synchrony created through social touch serves as a biological pathway in infant development, supporting infant learning and social bonding.

The perception of interpersonal touch is heavily influenced by its source. For example, a gentle stroke from a loved one is generally more pleasant than the same tactile stimulation from a stranger. A recent study (Aguirre et al., 2019) showed that infant heart rates decreased more in reaction to strokes from their caregiver vs. a stranger. The knowledge that interpersonal touch reduces infants' response to stress (Feldman et al., 2010) and enhances social learning (Della Longa et al., 2021) has become the basis for the development of therapeutic touch for infants and young children in stressful situations. A small sample study (Wong et al., 2013) examined the impact of therapeutic touch on children age 3–18 years old with pediatric cancer and found significant decreases in scores for pain, stress, and fatigue for participants and parents; caregivers' and parents' perception of their children's pain also decreased significantly.

The use of touch, and the quality and quantity of touch, is extremely personal. A child's touch preferences can vary from day to day and are also dependent on their reactions to specific treatments. Skin-to-skin contact, especially with very young babies, can be particularly soothing. Touch during MSDMT sessions includes gestural actions as simple as holding a child's hand with massaging strokes, stroking their forehead or scalp, covering them with a blanket, snuggling with their favorite plush toy, or placing cold or hot packs on areas the patient experiences as painful. Touch also includes specific massage strokes with one or both hands on particular areas of the body, the whole body, or having the patient sense their parent lying close to them. Touch can be used at the beginning of a session to calm the body and set a tone of relaxation; it can also be effective to soothe and dissipate pain when it arises.

There are many different massage techniques (Field, 2019). Though it's especially advantageous to have trained massage therapists administer these methods, there are some simple techniques that, with practice, can be performed by the caregiver. The most important guideline is to pay attention to the quality of touch related to the amount of pressure used; length of the stroke, timing, and how much of the body is being stroked at one time; and providing a single stroke or alternating strokes, such as gliding down the left and then the right leg. It is essential to notice how the child responds to varying qualities of pressure; adding and releasing pressure using rhythmic or flowing actions can be very soothing. The amount of pressure of the stroke is especially important (Field et al., 2010): Firm or deep touch calms and organizes the brain, whereas light touch is alerting; light touch must be administered with care because it can be experienced as tickling or tentative. Actions to explore include strokes with steady pressure, cupping your hand while creating clockwise or counterclockwise circular strokes on the abdomen, and long strokes down the legs continuing to the feet, alternating hands to create a sequential, continuous flowing experience.

Long strokes that integrate the painful area with other parts of the body can redirect the focus from the painful spot. Short, pressing strokes or pulsing in a squeeze-and-release rhythm can also be effective to target and break up these spots. Even massaging the extremities – such as the head, neck, or the feet – can soothe the whole body. If the child is especially sensitive to touch, or becomes uncomfortable with touch, placing our hands close to their body without touching enables the child to feel the energy and heat of touch and its soothing presence. Once it is clear that the baby senses us, we slowly and gently glide our hands in the air down their body, starting from the top of their head or torso. By moving slowly and pausing intermittently, we can sense the baby's energy and temperature changes. This may be all that is needed to calm the baby, or, after a few stokes, the baby may respond well to placing our hand on their body and letting it settle, taking in the sensation of our hand and our presence.

Through touch, we may also stimulate the proprioceptive and vestibular systems, layering several systems at one time. For example, when a baby expresses distress, we may lift her, placing her on our shoulder while stroking or patting her back. The vestibular system is stimulated as we move the baby through the air, changing her position from lying to upright; the proprioceptive system is aroused as we hold the baby, firmly providing full body-to-body contact. If we bounce or move around the room, the vestibular system is engaged again.

Proprioception

Proprioception is very closely linked with qualities of touch during MSDMT sessions. Simply stated, proprioception relates to how we sense our body's position in space. Through the proprioceptive system, we sense the location, position, orientation, and movement of our muscles and joints as they relate to different parts of our body while moving. It is activated through proprioceptors in our muscles, ligaments, tendons, and the periphery of our body sending information to our brain. It is an additional system that calms and organizes the brain. Pushing, pulling, jumping, and using muscles all engage proprioception; pressure does, too. Chewing, biting, and sucking all are oral proprioceptive sensations that work closely with taste, the gustatory sense, and are discussed in that section. During pain episodes, providing experiences that enable the child to press or push against your hand, the bed, or other sturdy object also stimulates proprioceptive feedback and redirects internal sensations outward. For young babies and toddlers, having the caregiver hold the child in what is known as a bucket seat – placing the baby's back against the front of the parent's body as the parent scoops their arms underneath the baby's knees – allows the infant's pelvis to be free while rocking, or swaying the baby in a rhythmic manner. This provides good proprioceptive feedback within the baby's torso and can release tension and holding, especially with abdominal and back pain.

Alternating pressure from one side of the body to the other – for example, by firmly stroking the left foot from the heel to the toes and starting the same stroke on the right heel as you leave the left toe – creates a circular rhythmic sensation that has a calming effect that can be felt through the whole body. Attuning the timing and quality of the pressure to the intensity and style of the patient's vocalizations creates a rhythmic embodied dialogue that can organize and stabilize the felt experience. As this multimodal interchange becomes established, entrainment is palpable, as the auditory and proprioceptive temporal rhythmic cues resonate between the therapist and the patient. Through this oscillating duet, the actions and vocalizations synchronize, slowing down and calming the child.

Vestibular

The vestibular system enables us to orient where our body is in space, contributing to our sense of balance, informing us about movement, vibration, and the position of our head in relationship to gravity. The vestibular receptors are located in the inner ear and are composed of three fluid-filled canals. This fluid moves when we move our head or sense gravitational force or shifts of movement in the environment. The semicircular canals coordinate with the neural areas of the brain that control our eye actions to maintain our upright position as we engage in actions and different postures. The horizontal canal detects rotation around the vertical axis, the anterior semicircular canal detects forward/backward planal movement, and the posterior canal senses frontal plane directionality. Depending on how it is activated, this system can be calming or arousing.

MSDMT activities that engage the vestibular system are very important in regulating the young patient's experience and creating a calming environment, because it is the unifying system in the brain, modifying and coordinating information received from the tactile, proprioceptive, visual, and auditory systems. Rolling, spinning, swinging, rocking, and bending all stimulate the vestibular receptors. When experiencing pain, babies and young patients often move parts or all of their whole bodies, vigorously throwing, thrashing, wiggling, and pressing. Engaging the patient in rocking actions prior to the onset of pain, such as swaying them from side to side, rocking them forward and backward or up and down, can create a continuous, mesmerizing, and comforting experience. Alternatively, developing an accented rhythmic beat directs the child's attention, creating a full-body sense of organization. This can override a focus on isolated areas they may be experiencing as painful. Direction, intensity, and whether an action is performed with an accented or even tempo will vary depending on the patient's level of discomfort. For example, the phrasing of the movement action can be performed as smooth; accented in a steady 4/4 count, or a 3/4 waltz count with the first beat accented. In intense discomfort, "drop and swing" actions while securely holding the child in a bucket seat pose or up on our shoulder can be especially helpful, providing a slight level change in space.

Upward/downward, side-to-side, or forward/backward actions all add different stimulations that can be helpful during painful episodes. Intensifying the rhythmic quality of the action in a mirroring, exaggerated manner by matching the patient's cry and then slowing down creates an organizing rhythmic focus that soothes the baby. Adding more pressure and body-to-body contact during the swing or rocking actions are additional ways to add or take away multisensory input. Slightly suspending the child's body away from the adult's torso while swaying elongates the spine takes pressure off their pelvis, and can be very relieving, as well. Holding the child's ankles, feet, knees, or pelvis while sending a gentle vibrational rocking up and down through their body, known as the heel rock, creates a rhythmic wave sensation that can also be very helpful (Bartenieff & Lewis, 1980). These positions provide a full-body sensation with less body-to-body contact. If the child cannot tolerate any touch, rocking the bed in this rhythmic manner is another option for creating an overall undulating sensation that is soothing and not intrusive.

Auditory

The auditory system is highly coordinated with the attuned toning verbal and vocal sensations discussed in interoception. Vocalizing in a manner that attunes to the quality of the child's cries creates a palpable flow, calming the patient as the auditory sensations resonate between the therapist and patient. As discussed in Chapter 10, music therapists use the term entrainment to describe the synchronous tonal flow that occurs when the frequency of the auditory/rhythmic pattern between two people is matched (Thaut et al., 2015). Attending to the quality and cadence of our voice and vocal tone also guides the child's experience away from focusing on the treatment and pain perception. Being playful and engaging in a captivating storytelling manner during guided-imagery scenarios also captures the child's attention. This is especially helpful when the child is experiencing a surge of pain, because the emphasis in our vocal tone can parallel the child's felt experience while simultaneously redirecting them away as they stay engaged in the felt-imagery of the story. Shifting to a more soothing, steady, even rhythm and a slower, almost monotonous, vocal quality can be helpful in creating a subtle hypnotic state and calming environment (Olness, 1996). Babies are particularly responsive to their parents' voices in talking and singing (Loewy, 2015); regardless of the quality of a parent's singing voice, it is helpful to encourage parents to talk and sing, especially if this is part of their bedtime ritual. This provides a sense of the parent's consistent presence and attention to the child, manifesting feelings of familiarity, normalcy, and safety during a time that feels so foreign.

As discussed in Chapter 10, the regular 80 bpm of lullabies can be particularly pacifying for babies (Friedman et al., 2010). Young babies are also universally soothed by female vocals (O'Callaghan, 2008). Adding recorded music can enhance the environment and create additional ways to engage the child. It is important to emphasize that all types of music can be helpful since music choices are very personal. Tortora learned this directly when one child she worked with used a construction truck soundtrack to accompany him during a difficult treatment. As she sensed the power of the machines digging vigorously into the depths of the earth, followed by the high-pitched beeping as the truck backed up, the grunting of gears hauling the dirt, and the large puff of mechanical "gas" released as the dirt was thrown and dropped onto tall mounds of earth, she had a visceral response that was fully captivating. It clearly transported them both to an intensely physical experience of strength throughout the treatment.

Live music-making by playing instruments can also add to the auditory experience. During the active parts of treatment, we use percussive instruments such as egg shakers, drums, and xylophones to match and release the intensity of feelings evoked by the anticipation and experience of the medical treatment. Shifting to an ocean drum or a rainstick creates a more soothing background environment, especially if it matches the quality and flow of the child's breath. Providing imagery that emulates the undulating ocean tides gliding in and out on the shore adds visual input to the experience. This often resets the tone of the room and simplifies the auditory stimulation, creating a rhythmic, rocking auditory experience. Limiting auditory input is especially common during more difficult periods of treatment, when the patient appears to be in a very heightened arousal state. Minimizing talking to the patient and reducing directives or questions so only one person is speaking can help the child maintain their focused meditative stance with less input to manage.

Visual

The visual system refers to both the therapist's keen observation of the child to assess their level of arousal and interactive engagement and the child's eye gaze. Especially with babies, eye gaze is one way they tell us if, how, and to what they are attending, and what behavior state they may be in. Are they fully awake and alert, or drowsy? Noticing if the baby is looking directly at the practitioner, their parent, looking away, focusing deeply on something else, or appearing to be in a dazed or unfocused state provides valuable information that can guide the next steps of the intervention. Direct visual contact may be soothing or may be overloading for the patient. Babies use gaze – looking and looking away – to regulate their visual input. Allowing the baby to ebb and flow their attention, by letting them direct how long they focus their attention, divert their focus, return their gaze, or even close their eyes, helps them feel a sense of agency and self-organization.

The timing and intensity of the adults' facial expressions of warmth or playfulness can also shift a child's mood and ease. Does the child benefit from being distracted by a plush toy or an electronic device? Adjusting the lighting can change the environment, as well. Additional visual props we use include multicolored light beams, rainbow streamers, and colorful scarves that float and flow to guide visual attention. At these young ages, electronic props and online programs are used minimally; maintaining live interpersonal connections are preferable to build the child's social/emotional systems of support.

Olfactory

The olfactory system can be added in subtle and more obvious ways. Some children become highly sensitive to scent and cannot tolerate it during treatments. Very young babies are deeply attuned to the scent of their primary caregivers, so having articles of clothing with their parents' scent to snuggle with is soothing, helping the baby sense their parent's presence, even if they are not able to be physically present. It is also remarkable how effective it can be for a toddler to cuddle with their favorite plush toy. Adding essential oils like lavender, on its own or in a cream gently massaged on the child, can also be very soothing. Though aromatherapy, a holistic healing treatment that uses aromatic oils to enhance physical and emotional health, goes beyond the scope of this book, on a very simple level, it can be successful in changing the atmosphere of the room, deeply calming the child and the parent (PDQ® Integrative, 2021).

Taste

Taste, the final sensory system discussed here, is the least common system employed during treatments because many procedures limit food intake prior to and during procedures. However, when possible, this sense – especially when combined with biting, sucking, and chewing, which are all oral proprioceptive sensations – can be very organizing, having a calming effect on the brain and whole body. Nursing or bottle-feeding an infant in a warm embrace is very regulating and supports the emotional relationship. When children perform non-nutritive actions, such as chewing, biting, sucking, and swallowing, they are giving themselves intense proprioceptive input in an attempt to self-regulate. This may include sucking on their thumb, finger, pacifier, collar, or sleeve. The rhythmic sensation created by sucking provides deep sensory input. Tastes and flavors are also stimulating and organizing: sour, spicy, bitter, or minty flavors; textures such as chewy, crunchy, and mushy. Sipping a cool drink can provide a refreshing internal sensation that resets focus in the moment, while having a soothing effect on the body and brain.

Conclusion

The MSDMT approach creates an environment of emotional safety and security for the young pediatric patient, sensed on both emotional and neurological levels. Understanding that difficult experiences may be somaticized and held in the child's implicit memory, the dance therapist responds to the verbal and nonverbal cues of the child to create a multisensory atmosphere of engagement to soothe the child. Placing primary importance on the concept that early-life experiences with significant caregivers are at the core of security, parents play key roles in implementing the multisensory-based activities. By creating an embodied experience of attuned listening, loving support, and coping, it is our hope that we are helping the child and parent navigate the paradox that sometimes healing hurts, and facilitating memories of resilience and strength through embracing, caring relationships with the whole treatment team.

References

Aguirre, M., Couderc, A., Epinat-Duclos, J., & Mascaro, O. (2019). Infants discriminate the source of social touch at stroking speeds eliciting maximal firing rates in CT-fibers. *Developmental Cognitive Neuroscience, 36*, 100639–100639. https://doi.org/10.1016/j. dcn.2019.100639

Bartenieff, I., & Lewis, D. (1980). *Body movements: Coping with the environment.* Gordon and Breach Science Publishers.

Charlton, J. E. (2005). *Core curriculum for professional edcuation in pain.* IASP Press.

Della Longa, L., Dragovic, D., & Farroni, T. (2021). In touch with the heartbeat: Newborn's cardiac sensitivity to affective and non affective touch. *International Journal of Environmental Research and Public Health, 18*(5), 2212.

Denworth, L. (2015, July–August). The social power of touch. *Scientific American Mind, 26*(4), 30–39.

Dunbar, R. I. (2010, February). The social role of touch in humans and primates: Behavioural function and neurobiological mechanisms. *Neuroscience and Biobehavioral Reviews, 34*(2), 260–268. https://doi.org/10.1016/j.neubiorev.2008.07.001

Feldman, R. (2011). Maternal touch and the developing infant. In H. Matthew & W. Sandra (Eds.), *The handbook of touch: Neuroscience, behavioral, and health perspectives* (pp. 373–408). Springer.

Feldman, R., Singer, M., & Zagoory, O. (2010). Touch attenuates infant's physiological reactivity to stress. *Development Science, 13*(2), 271–278.

Field, T. (2014). *Touch.* MIT Press.

Field, T. (2019). Pediatric massage therapy research: A narrative review. *Children, 6*(6), 78. www.mdpi.com/2227-9067/6/6/78

Field, T., Diego, M., & Hernandez-Reif, M. (2010, May). Moderate pressure is essential for massage therapy effects. *International Journal of Neuroscience, 120*(5), 381–385. https://doi. org/10.3109/00207450903579475

Fogel, A. (2009). *The psychophysiology of self-awareness: Rediscovering the lost art of body sense.* W. W. Norton.

Friedman, S., Kaplan, R., Rosenthal, M., & Console, P. (2010). Music therapy in perinatal psychiatry: Use of lullabies for pregnant and postpartum women with mental illness. *Music and Medicine, 2*(4), 219–225.

Gaensbauer, T. (1995). Trauma in the preverbal period. Symptoms, memories, and developmental impact. *Psychoanal Study Child, 50*, 122–149.

Gaensbauer, T. (2004). Telling their stories: Representation and reenactment of traumatic experiences occurring in the first year of life. *Zero to Three, 24*(5), 25–31.

Khalsa, S. S., Adolphs, R., Cameron, O. G., Critchley, H. D., Davenport, P. W., Feinstein, J. S., Feusner, J. D., Garfinkel, S. N., Lane, R. D., Mehling, W. E., Meuret, A. E., Nemeroff, C. B., Oppenheimer, S., Petzschner, F. H., Pollatos, O., Rhudy, J. L., Schramm, L. P., Simmons, W. K., Stein, M. B., Stephan, K. E., Van den Bergh, O., Van Diest, I., von Leupoldt, A., Paulus, M. P., Ainley, V., Al Zoubi, O., Aupperle, R., Avery, J., Baxter, L., Benke, C., Berner, L., Bodurka, J., Breese, E., Brown, T., Burrows, K., Cha, Y.-H., Clausen, A., Cosgrove, K., Deville, D., Duncan, L., Duquette, P., Ekhtiari, H., Fine, T., Ford, B., Garcia Cordero, I., Gleghorn, D., Guereca, Y., Harrison, N. A., Hassanpour, M., Hechler, T., Heller, A., Hellman, N., Herbert, B., Jarrahi, B., Kerr, K., Kirlic, N., Klabunde, M., Kraynak, T., Kriegsman, M., Kroll, J., Kuplicki, R., Lapidus, R., Le, T., Hagen, K. L., Mayeli, A., Morris, A., Naqvi, N., Oldroyd, K., Pané-Farré, C., Phillips,

R., Poppa, T., Potter, W., Puhl, M., Safron, A., Sala, M., Savitz, J., Saxon, H., Schoenhals, W., Stanwell-Smith, C., Teed, A., Terasawa, Y., Thompson, K., Toups, M., Umeda, S., Upshaw, V., Victor, T., Wierenga, C., Wohlrab, C., Yeh, H.-W., Yoris, A., Zeidan, F., Zotev, V., & Zucker, N. (2018, June 1). Interoception and mental health: A roadmap. *Biological Psychiatry: Cognitive Neuroscience and Neuroimaging, 3*(6), 501–513. https://doi.org/https://doi.org/10.1016/j.bpsc.2017.12.004

Lee, D., Serrano, V., von Schulz, J., Fields, D., & Buchholz, M. (2021). From patients to partners: Promoting health equity in pediatric primary care with the healthysteps program. *Zero to Three, 42*(2), 72–78.

Lieberman, A. (2021, March 8). *Promoting child-parent symbolic play to repair early trauma.* The Spectrum of Play, Online Conference. https://profectum.org/2021-conference-spectrum-play/

Loewy, L. (2015). NICU music therapy: Song of kin as critical lullaby in research and practice. *Annals of the New York Academy of Sciences, 1337*(The Neurosciences and Music V), 178–185. https://doi.org/10.1111/nyas.12648

Mahler, K. (2017). *Interoception: The eighth sensory system.* AAPC Publishing.

Morrison, I., Löken, L. S., & Olausson, H. (2010, July). The skin as a social organ. *Experimental Brain Research, 204*(3), 305–314. https://doi.org/10.1007/s00221-009-2007-y

Nguyen, T., Abney, D. H., Salamander, D., Bertenthal, B. I., & Hoehl, S. (2021, December 1). Proximity and touch are associated with neural but not physiological synchrony in naturalistic mother-infant interactions. *NeuroImage, 244*, 118599. https://doi.org/https://doi.org/10.1016/j.neuroimage.2021.118599

O'Callaghan, C. (2008, April–May). Lullament: Lullaby and lament therapeutic qualities actualized through music therapy. *American Journal of Hospice & Palliative Care, 25*(2), 93–99. https://doi.org/10.1177/1049909107310139

Olness, K. (1996). *Hypnosis and hypnotherapy with children.* Gilford.

PDQ® Integrative, A., & Complementary Therapies Editorial Board. (2021, October 25, 2019). *PDQ aromatherapy with essential oils.* National Cancer Institute. Retrieved March 21, 2021, from www.cancer.gov/about-cancer/treatment/cam/hp/aromatherapy-pdq

Porges, S. W., & Daniel, S. (2017). Play and dynamics of treating pediatric medical trauma. In S. Daniel & C. Trevarthen (Eds.), *Rhythms of relating in children's therapies: Connecting creatively with vunerable children* (pp. 113–124). Jessica Kingsley Publishers.

Stern, D. (1985). *The interpersonal world of the infant.* Basic Books, Inc.

Thaut, M., McIntosh, G., & Hoemberg, V. (2015, February 18). Neurobiological foundations of neurologic music therapy: Rhythmic entrainment and the motor system [Review]. *Frontiers in Psychology, 5*(1185). https://doi.org/10.3389/fpsyg.2014.01185

Tobin, D. (2011). The anatomy and physiology of skin. In M. Hertenstein & S. Weiss (Eds.), *The handbook of touch: Neuroscience, behavioral, and health perspectives* (pp. 3–32). Springer Publishing Company.

Tortora, S. (2006). *The dancing dialogue: Using the communicative power of movement with young children.* Paul H. Brookes Publishing Company.

Tortora, S. (2016). Dance movement psychotherapy in early childhood treatment and in pediatric oncology. In S. W. Chaiklin (Ed.), *The art and science of dance/movement therapy: Life is dance* (2nd ed., pp. 159–181). Routledge.

Tortora, S. (2019). Children are born to dance! Pediatric medical dance/movement therapy: The view from integrative pediatric oncology. *Children, 6*(14), 1–27. https://doi.org/10.3390/children6010014

Vincent, S. R., Tortora, S., Shaw, J., Basiner, J., Devereaux, C., Mulcahy, S., & Ponsini, M. (2007). Collaborating with a mission: The andrea rizzo foundation spreads the gift of dance/movement therapy. *American Journal of Dance Therapy*, *29*(1), 51–58.

Wong, J., Ghiasuddin, A., Kimata, C., Patelesio, B., & Siv, A. (2013). The impact of healing touch on pediatric oncology patient. *Integrative Cancer Therapies*, *12*(1), 25–30.

Chapter 12

Summary of Key Points

This chapter is a synthesis of the information provided in this book, summarizing our joint dance/movement therapy and child psychiatry approach in the assessment and the treatment of very young children with life-threatening illness and their parents/caregivers during and after medical treatment.

Early illness – especially when life threatening – can have a profound effect on all developmental stages of growth, continuing into childhood, adolescence, and adulthood. The intrinsic body, movement, and nonverbal aspects of dance/movement therapy, coupled with the very young child's natural propensity for creative expressive dance and movement, uniquely position dance/movement therapy as an effective treatment method that can support a child to synthesize potentially traumatic aspects of their medical experience as they undergo treatment. The aesthetic and expressive elements of dance/movement activities support the patient to create new dynamic patterns, linking motor actions, interoceptive sensations, perceptions, affect and memories, with the potential to shape new cognitive understandings, memories, and felt experiences. The key practical points of our assessment and therapeutic approaches are summarized in what follows.

Goals

Provide young patients with a way to explore their experience to develop a sense of agency during treatment and create an embodied, coherent narrative of their experience.

•

Teach parents how to attune to their baby's nonverbal actions to enable the baby to feel his actions have been heard and are communicative.

•

Support adjustment and acceptance of the child's body rather than focusing on the dysfunctions caused by the disease.

• ■ •

DOI: 10.4324/9781003134800-13

Goals *(cont.)*

Strive to create an environment that preserves both the developing parent–infant relationship and the baby's psyche-soma experience.

•

Increase the parent's sense of competence in parenting and caring for their child during illness.

•

Support the caregiver's emotional availability especially during frightening or pain-related interventions, to keep the experience tolerable and foster a supportive caregiver–infant relationship.

•

Provide a felt experience of consistent attuned support with a familiar caregiver/medical professional, especially during procedures that the infant may perceive as uncomfortable or painful, to build the infant's embodied experience, supporting the development of later regulatory strategies and skills.

•

Create a secure relationship with the parents to increase their awareness of their own projections and nonverbal behaviors linked to difficult or traumatic experiences related to their child's illness that are challenging to express and may influence their current parenting.

Key Questions to Keep in Mind During Treatment

How does a baby's medical illness inform and affect the baby's experience of his body in the formulation of self?

•

How does the baby incorporate sensations that inhibit smooth bodily functioning and movement exploration, at the very least, and create felt perceptions that are painful and potentially life-threatening, at worst?

•

How does the intrusion of medically necessary procedures, performed outside of the baby's own exploratory and willful actions, contribute to the maturing psychological, cognitive, and sensational self?

•

How does the infant's exposure to bright lights, noxious odors, loud and uncomfortable auditory stimuli, temperature fluctuations, abrasive tactile sensations, and other multisensory factors inform his psyche-soma experience?

• ■ •

Key Questions to Keep in Mind During Treatment *(cont.)*

What are the impacts on the young child's mind, body, and spirit when illness and treatment leave the young child impaired?

•

How can we best support the parents/caregivers during treatment, so they can create an embodied sense of safety for the young patient, being fully present for their child during difficult moments, and helping their child reach a calm state after treatment?

•

How can the child and the caregivers be helped to discuss their unspeakable experiences of illness, pain, and/or fear of death?

Factors to Keep in Mind When Engaging with the Child and Their Parents/Caregivers to Support Psyche-Soma Development

Young Child

Keeping the young child's felt embodied experience in the forefront during a complex medical illness is essential.

•

Babies' social and emotional development, as it is expressed through their embodied experiences, must be considered side by side with medical treatment.

•

The "sense of body" concept postulates that the baby's early body-based experiences shape how she communicates, explores, and organizes intrapersonal and interpersonal experiences.

•

We don't have to wait until infants have verbal skills for them to feel they are good communicators regarding their medical experience.

•

Responding to a baby's nonverbal communication empowers even the youngest patients as they experience their expressive actions prompting attuned responses from adults.

•

Babies remember pain and consequently react differently to subsequent painful experiences. Anticipatory stress with recurrent painful procedures needs to be considered.

• ■ •

Factors to Keep in Mind When Engaging with the Child and Their Parents/Caregivers to Support Psyche-Soma Development *(cont.)*

Behaviors include the following.
- Withdrawal.
- Increased irritability.
- Extreme anxiety and clinging.
- Muteness.

•

Signs of pain in infants with critical illness can be subtle, including the following.
- Imperceptible movement.
- Sudden gaze change.
- Vigilant gaze, frozen facial expressions, extreme body stillness.
- Unresponsive to distraction attempts.

•

Painful experiences during some medical treatments are inevitable. A better predictor of the effect of the experience, and whether coping skills are developing, is the baby's specific responses to being soothed and his ability to be comforted. Children who take an active coping role and are more cooperative with hospital staff show less disturbance after discharge.

•

Children in the first three years of life are more vulnerable to toxic stress, but they are also more sensitive to the positive impact of early interventions.

•

Babies can be reoriented to soothe from overstimulation/distress through interpersonal interactions that promote emotional social connections.

Parent/Caregiver–Child Relationship

Caregivers act as a bridge, providing the embodied experience of redirected attention.

•

Electronic devices are often used to replace this important emotional social experience. Being selective about when to use electronic devices is essential to not undermining/interrupting the effectiveness of the developing attachment relationship, self-coping skills, and emotional social development.

• ■ •

**Factors to Keep in Mind When Engaging
with the Child and Their Parents/Caregivers
to Support Psyche-Soma Development** *(cont.)*

The parent/caregiver's emotional availability is an essential
component of the young child's ability to process their medical
experience. A serious pediatric illness may compromise the
parent's availability and unconsciously undermine the infant's
sense of self.

•

The Embodied Parenting program is used to teach parents how
to attend to their baby's and their own nonverbal cues to support
self-regulation and co-regulation, supporting the attachment
relationship. It provides parents with culturally sensitive dance,
movement, and music activities to soothe and engage babies, aiding
their developing attachment relationship.

•

The DANCE tool provides a way to determine and understand
specific nonverbal qualities that influence the dynamics of the
parent/caregiver–child relationship.

•

Whatever the method of working on the parent–infant relationship
is, assessment of the infant's characteristics, as well as the caregivers'
own history of traumas and pain-related experiences, are necessary
for planning the intervention. Research shows that there is a
reciprocal relationship between infant and parent behaviors when
evaluating infant pain.

•

Factors demonstrating parental resilience include the following.
• Parents' perception of the disease.
• Personal competence.
• Self-confidence.
• Acceptance of change.
• Self-control.
• Secure existing relationships –
the quality of the parental dyadic relationship
and each partner's coping styles.

•

Planning for the intervention should be based on the
assessment of the infant's and the caregivers' strengths,
weaknesses, and the DC: 0–5 multiaxial diagnostic
formulation of the whole clinical situation.

• • •

Factors to Keep in Mind When Engaging with the Child and Their Parents/Caregivers to Support Psyche-Soma Development *(cont.)*

Long-Term Impact of Serious Medical Illness

Caregivers are often surprised when their healthy child creates a new set of anxieties and parenting issues, including the following.
• Difficulties in setting limits and appropriate behavioral expectations.
• Inability to relax with the thought and belief that their child is well.

Behaviors and symptoms that may appear post-treatment include the following.
• Tantrums.
• Social anxiety, especially with adults.
• Difficultly engaging with siblings and peers.
• Attentional and regulatory difficulties.
• Learning differences.
• Fears.
• Anxiety.
• Depression.
• Obsessive/compulsive behaviors.
• Delays achieving developmental milestones including self-care and toileting.
• Eating disorders.
• Issues related to family dynamics.

Support the Young Child's Embodied Experience to Create a Sense of Agency

See Appendix C for a detailed handout about ways to understand and engage with baby's nonverbal cues.
•
Attunement – match or complement the nonverbal quality of a young child's movements but not duplicating actions.
•
Mirroring – match a child's mood, facial expressions, and exact actions.

• ■ •

Support the Young Child's Embodied
Experience to Create a Sense of Agency *(cont.)*

Note when baby's behaviors are an emotional expression
for engagement vs. when they are an attempt to self-
regulate and additional input is dysregulating.

•

Baby/toddler-centered care includes constancy from
home to hospital to home. Include rituals from home as
much as possible during hospitalizations.

•

Support parents' needs, creating a welcoming
environment for them to focus on their own emotions,
and support their ability to be a calm presence for their
child.

xxxxxxxxxxxxxxxxxxxxxxxxxxxxxxxxxxxxxxxxxxxxxxxxxxxxxxxxxxxxxxxxxx

During Medical Procedures, *When Possible*

xxxxxxxxxxxxxxxxxxxxxxxxxxxxxxxxxxxxxxxxxxxxxxxxxxxxxxxxxxxxxxxxxx

Take note of the feeling tone of the environment, adjust
lighting and sounds, and take away overwhelming
distractions to create a soothing/engaging environment
that appeals to the child's interests to focus their
attention.

•

Describe to the child (at all ages) what you are about to
do, and pause to let the child take it in.

•

Pace medical treatments by adding pauses to attune to
the child's reactions. Pausing and pacing a procedure
enables a moment of adjustment for the child.

•

Have the parent/caregiver provide a solely pacifying
presence, letting the medical team administer the
treatment.

•

Specific soothing behaviors depend on the child's
requests and nonverbal responses. These may include the
following.
• Providing eye contact or no eye contact.
• Calming voice/singing/storytelling/praying/chanting/
vocal toning.

• • •

Support the Young Child's Embodied Experience to Create a Sense of Agency *(cont.)*

• Redirecting the child's attention with visual/auditory distractions, active play, holding a plush toy or blanket.
• Calmly embracing the child while attuning your breath patterns.
• Embracing the child post-treatment until calm.

When parents are not available

• Reassure the child of his primary caregiver's love and care, even in their absence.
• When possible, have consistent caregivers from the medical team present as a primary comforting, emotionally supportive presence.

Steps to Establish Nonverbal Connection

Learn the baby's specific nonverbal cues of engagement and distress to be able to anticipate their reactions and prevent stress and dysregulation. Embodied countertransference: become aware of your own nonverbal cues, and the child's reactions to you, to optimize your engagement and avoid creating frightened responses from the baby. See Appendix D for simple activities.

Eye Gaze and Facial Expressivity

Establish comfortable joint attention through visual engagement leaving room for child's ebb and flow of attention and expression.

• Be available for eye contact when the infant is seeking social connection.
• Avoid soliciting eye contact that usurps the infant's capacity to set the pace.
• Share in infant's delight with your own facial expressivity when initiated by the infant.

• ■ •

Steps to Establish Nonverbal Connection *(cont.)*

• Detect signs of sadness or vigilance in expression or
eye gaze, e.g. blank gaze, flat affect, lack of vitality in
expression. Wonder about their potential significance/
message in the context of the child's overall experience.
Note how often child visually references parent while
engaging with you.

Regulation of Body and Mood

Attend to the child's presenting behavioral state, mood,
arousal threshold, and activity level before engaging.
Pause, also noting the overall tone in the room as well,
adapting your own mood/tone to complement or support
the family.

•

Supportive regulatory, relaxing, and/or engaging
activities include breath awareness that attunes to the
child's breathing pattern and the use of carefully layered
multisensory activities, paying attention to how the child
responds to each sensory modality.

•

Nonverbal cues that determine the child's mood include
the following.

• Activity level.
• Arousal/amount of input needed to engage.
• Facial expressions.
• Emotional reactivity.
• Tone of vocal expression.
• Distress response to limitations.
• Response to frustration.
• Soothability.
• Quality of alert responsiveness and orienting behaviors.
• Reaction to touch.
• Body proximity (where child places body in relation to par-
ent and you to maintain engagement), e.g. does child need to
touch or be held by parent to engage with you?

• ■ •

Steps to Establish Nonverbal Connection *(cont.)*

Prosody

Pay attention to the quality of your vocal tone, using your voice to make an emotional connection. Babies respond most to infant-directed speech and infant-directed singing. Matching your vocal pattern to the baby's vocalizations and actions will focus their attention and stimulate their curiosity.

Build Trust Nonverbally

Through the quality of your body-to-body communication and caring touch:

- Notice your muscular tension and breath pattern before coming closer or engaging in physical contact.
- Pick up the baby only when they strongly signal this desire by reading their specific nonverbal cues.
- Adjust your physical stance to attune to the child's non-verbal reactions, such as engaging at the child's eye level and posture.
- Touch as a form of communication. Loving (parental) touch, and skin-to-skin care in humans, has an organizing effect on the baby's stress system.

Rhythm and Melody

These can have a regulatory function organizing the environment. Pay attention to the pace and rhythmic qualities in your nonverbal and verbal interactions. Use dance/movement games with rhythm and melody to create a playful give-and-take dancing dialogue.
Use rhythm to soothe the baby by holding and rocking them, prior to, during, or after a painful or scary procedure. Providing external rhythmic support attuning to child's cry/vocal distress through your voice and/or vocal toning can organize and soothe the child.

• ■ •

Steps to Establish Nonverbal Connection (*cont.*)

Self-Discovery

Provide opportunities for the baby to explore their bodily self through their own movement explorations, rather than anticipating their actions and doing it for them. For example: when the baby wants a toy just out of their grasp, support them to shift their weight forward and reach for it, rather than handing it to them.

Object Permanence

Support emotional connection through dyadic play using varying spatial distances and dance-play fingerplay games, including peek-a-boo, hide and seek, and scarf play.

Enhance Relating

Through dance/movement activities and dance-play, fingerplay and action songs that include attunement, mirroring, turn-taking, and follow the leader. For examples, see Appendix D.

Support Movement and Motor Exploration

Create a sense of agency by supporting the child's own exertion and initiations to experience their own body/ movement efforts while exploring developmental movement patterns, five fundamental actions, and creative dance-play.

Independence

Support the child's own movement-based initiatives and individuality by providing opportunities for solo dance explorations with adults as the audience, and support independent creative craft, physical play, and building/construction toys beyond electronic devices and TV.

Sensory/Full-Body Regulation and Play

Instruments for Rhythm, Engagement, and Soothing

- Egg shakers.
- Ocean drum.
- Buffalo drum.
- Chimes.
- Rainstick.
- Tone bar.
- Xylophone.
- Gato box.
- Recorded music: rhymes, lullabies, pop, classical, ambient, child's/parent's favorites, culturally specific.

Resistive objects to pull, push, cuddle, hide, cocoon in

Lycra fabric bands and tunnels, body sock, bungee cord, weighted vests/blankets/animals of assorted sizes, textured fabrics, blankets, and pillows.

Fidget and sensory manipulatives

Push pop-it bubble toys, glitter balls, bubbles, pinwheels, Play-Doh/clay, stretchy toy figures, marbles, jacks, scented hand cream, sand, and water.

Dance props

Sheer colorful scarves, rainbow streamers, tutus and skirts, masks, capes, hats, and crowns.

Active play

Speed spiral; balls of all sizes materials, and weights; swords; foam tubes; flashlights; building construction toys.

Obstacle course materials

Slide, glide, climb, swing: steps, slides, tunnels, scooters, yoga balls, balance beam, trapeze, Lycra hammock, rope, and mini-trampoline.

Arts and crafts

Drawing materials, child scissors, felt and other sewing materials, stickers, glitter, and glue.

Pretend play

Dress-up costumes, pretend food, tea sets, dishes, cookware, and baby dolls with blankets and bottles.

Action figures, animal figures, and family groupings

All sizes, including "scary" and "cuddly" figures (butterfly, dinosaur, bear, lion, snake, horse, giraffe); water/sea (shark, whale, octopus, crocodile); fantasy (unicorn, Pegasus, mermaid, merman).

Emotions and stories

Feeling charts, books, poems, story writing pads, and sandtrays.

Toys

Medical kits, cars, ambulances, child's own toys, blankets, stuffed animals, and dolls.

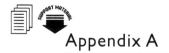

DANCE Tool

Outline of key nonverbal parameters of the opening vignette of Chapter 9, describing interaction between Adele [A] and Tortora [ST], who entered room when Adele was watching iPad without Mom present. The numbering of each sub-delineation (e.g. 1.1, 2.1) corresponds to each section of the vignette as it progresses. Tortora's observations on a body–mind–emotional level are labeled using the following terms: body = kinesthetic seeing (KE); mind = witnessing (W); emotion = kinesthetic empathy (KS). See Tortora (2006, 2013) for in-depth description and further case examples of these terms.

1. **Body**

   1.1 [A] Torso initially alert rolling weight side to side, driven by limbs flailing. [ST] Waiting at bedside with whole torso still, limbs at side, attuning to personal breath flow. (KS) Sensing need to slow and calm my whole body; (W) Create a calm, available presence before approaching further; (KE) Create compassionate and understanding emotionally embodied stance.

   1.2 [A] Torso held, erect and tight, with limbs at her sides when Adele is initially placed on up onto my shoulder. [ST] Maintain my vertical body stance with keen attention to maintaining organized aligned posture, and firmness in my arms. (KS) Create strong safe embrace.

   1.3 [A] In response to the vertical rhythmic rocking, her torso and limbs begin to slightly soften and ultimately she rests her head on the curve of my shoulder. When I shift the action to a side-to-side sway she adjusts and softens her whole body even more. [ST] I maintain my vertical alignment and wrap my arms around her torso as she adjusts on my shoulder. (W) Continue to make small adjustments in my body so that she feels my warm responsive presence.

2. **Facial Expressivity and Quality of Eye Gaze**

   2.1 [A] Eye contact avoidant; crying grimacing expression. [ST] Calm facial expression with soft direct eye contact. (KE) Creating warm expression, available without being overwhelming.

2.2   [A] Continues to avoid eye contact and gaze becomes fixed out into space without seeming to focus on anything specifically. [ST] Soften facial expression, eye gaze toward Adele, over my shoulder without direct gaze so as not to overwhelm her.

2.3   [A] As she rests her head in my shoulder, she turns her gaze toward me, and her face becomes increasingly peaceful. [ST] Now I orient my gaze toward her as best as I can and smile gently. (KE) I feel a deep sense of peace, calm and connection to Adele.

3.   Body Shapes

3.1   [A] While rolling torso is alert and contained appearing stiff except for limbs projecting making sporadic arc-like actions. [ST] Torso vertical, limbs a side and slight forward lean from waist upward. Breathing pattern creates shape-flow in upper torso/chest. (KS) Maintaining a contained less intrusive presence.

3.2   [A] Upper body pulled away from my torso as if attempting to push off of me with neck and head very vertically aligned with upper spine. [ST] While bending over to pick up Adele, maintaining a strong tilted vertical stance. Once upright again, stay vertically aligned, focusing more deeply on the flow of my breath and shaping my body gently to accommodate to her form. (W) Need to maintain quiet presence and layer in more sensory stimulation in slow manner. Pause verbalizations to give Adele time to adjust to our body-to-body contact. (KS) Attempting to create a soft physical contact for Adele to slowly relax into.

3.3   [A] Her body shapes into my torso, becoming heavier as she relaxes. [ST] I continue to adjust the shape of my body to accommodate to her adjustments. (W) I want to maintain a strong safe physical presence so that she can fully relax.

4.   Interactional Space

4.1   [A] Rolling from the middle to the side of her crib, back and forth, in her own (kinespheric) space separate from dance therapist. [ST] Pause, standing more than arm's-length away from the crib in (general) space with slight leaning forward of upper body, while still arm's-length away from crib. (W) I want Adele to know that I am here but that I will pace my approach to avoid physically bombarding her.

4.2   [A], [ST] Movement through space to reach close proximity, body-to-body contact.

4.3   [A], [ST] We slowly begin to move around the room as we transition to swaying. (W) We create a dancing dialogue through the room.

5. **Quality of Movement Actions**

5.1 [A] Quickness, pulsing, bound tension, strength in vocal tone of cry. [ST] Stillness, subtle direct focus, small slow actions. (KE) Maintain emotional steadiness and calm physical, emotional, and vocal tone.

5.2 [A] Increased bound tension in whole body, as if torso and limbs are all one unit. [ST] Slowness with slight increase and decrease of timing, strong arms, and soft chest/rib cage with more free flow through breath.

5.3 [A] Softening of her tension into a relative heaviness as she continues to relax. [ST] Using a slightly strong, direct and accelerated pulse during the rocking up and down to add rhythmic pulse, transitioning to a more undulating, fluid, and decelerated rhythm during the lullaby song. (KS) I feel my own body soften more as I attune to her gradual shifting into less tension. I feel a sense of synchrony as we both shift our physical state. (KE) I have become calmer, too.

6. **Quality and Frequency of Touch**

6.1 [A] Physical sensation of torso rolling on bed. [ST] Arms at side, sensing vertical stance and flow of breath. (W) Purposefully waiting before physically engaging Adele.

6.2 [A] Upper chest pulled away from my shoulders, arms legs and lower torso in contact with my torso. [ST] Maintaining firm hold with arms for security, while taking long steady breaths. (KS) Hoping Adele will feel the expansion and softening inward as I inhale and exhale.

6.3 [A] Increasing her body-to-body contact as she softens her whole torso into my body and rests her head into the curve of my shoulder. [ST] Maintaining the firm hold of my arms and soft flow of my breath as we dance up and down, and then around the room.

7. **Tempo and Phrasing of Nonverbal Style**

7.1 [A] Rapid rhythmic pulsing phrase to cry and rolling actions. [ST] Creating stillness with whole body, except for subtle slow flow of breath. When speaking, create even tempo with evenly paced, intermittent pauses. (W) Need to stay calm to balance her upset.

7.2 [A] Holding her body and breath while steadily pushing back. [ST] When bending down to pick up Adele, using slow consistent actions without qualitative variation. Once upright, pause, (W) provide Adele with a chance to adjust to our close contact.

7.3   [A] As her crying ceases, she begins to breathe in a softer regular rhythm with slightly longer duration of each breath. The pattern of her breath is complimentary to mine. [ST] At first, I match Adele's breath by pacing mine, and then shift into a rhythm that coordinates with hers but is slower, creating a half-time rhythm. (W) I want her to have a felt experience of a calmer regulated embodied state.

8. Vocal Patterns

8.1   [A] Crying with a strong pulsing pattern. [ST] Focus on slow calm breath pattern, slowly paced vocal tone with intermittent pausing. (W) Attempting to match Adele's crying pattern by modifying my breath to mirror hers, slowing it to match her in half-time.

9. Regulation/Co-Regulation

9.1   [A] Crying behavioral state: highly aroused and active motoric state through limbs and torso with some organization within flinging actions. [ST] Using breath and slow actions to maintain self-regulation, synchronizing breath pattern to compliment Adele's cries and actions. (KS) Sensing Adele's actions through my embodied breathing sensations.

9.2   [A] Shifting to fussy then active alert state: softening her cry while maintaining a regular rhythm. [ST] Continue with breath awareness and synchronizing with Adele's cries. (W) Pacing my actions to match Adele's actions to provide a felt-sensation of containment rather than escalation.

9.3   [A] Shifting into awake state: a more self-regulated organization of her physiological and emotional state is achieved as Adele calms her body and relaxes on my shoulder. [ST] I provide a clear calm state for Adele to sense through our close contact, supporting her ability to slow her own body down. As she calms, I realize that I, too, am relaxing my own highly attuned alert state, achieving co-regulation as we sway to the calming music.

10. Coherence

10.1   Though it is not clear yet how much Adele is aware of my presence, I am interpreting Adele's vocalizations and actions as a path to achieve more self-regulation, for although not engaging with me yet and crying, she is not withdrawn. Interpreting this as a potential to create a co-regulatory state by continuing to contingently respond, I feel confident to proceed by increasing our engagement.

10.2 Adele is becoming more aware of my support. I continue to create a calm, active presence as I respond to the shifts in her nonverbal actions.

10.3 Through the interactive dynamic engagement, Adele and I are able to shift into a coherent state facilitating both self- and co-regulated states and creating a harmonious "whole" as we sway to the lullaby music.

Reference

Tortora, S. (2006). *The dancing dialogue: Using the communicative power of movement with young children*. Paul H. Brookes Publishing Company.

Tortora, S. (2013). The essential role of the body in the parent-infant relationship: Nonverbal analysis of attachment. In J. F. Bettmann (Ed.), *Attachment-based clinical social work with children and adolescents* (pp. 141–164). Springer.

Appendix B

Example of an MSDMT Session Plan Using the Body–Mind–Emotional Continuum with an Infant or Toddler

I. **Check-in**. Discuss plan options prior to start of the treatment with the parent. Ask what elements of their bedtime ritual can be incorporated into this soothing routine, especially including songs, music, and holding positions. Try out elements of the plan prior to the medical treatment having the parent administer the activities, as well.

II. **Body**

    a. Layering senses.

        i. Visual options:

            1. Animated facial expressions.
            2. Adjust lighting.
            3. Determine amount and specific electronic devise use.
            4. Light beam play.
            5. Scarves or other props to stimulate visual focus.
            6. Notice the child's level of comfort with eye contact.

        ii. Interoception:

            1. Notice the flow of the child's breath; notice your breath flow; attune the flow of your breath to compliment the child's breath pattern; e.g. with infants, inhale to child's every one complete breath (inhale-exhale).
            2. Often the child is highly sensitive especially when perceiving pain.

                a. Add a hot/cold pack to the area of pain.
                b. If the child experiences pressure as if needing to use the toilet:

                    i. Put a diaper on the child to ease worry.
                    ii. If it is a sensation but not a real need, redirect the child's attention to pushing with their legs, arms, and/or feet against the bed, or against the parent's or dance therapist's hands/body.

3. Use of breath:

    a. Practice breathing games prior to prepare for the progression of symptoms during treatment.

        i. Inhale for three counts, pause, exhale for four counts.

        ii. Add pausing between the inhale and exhale breath in pretending to smell a flower, exhale and blow out a candle.

        iv. Blow bubbles to practice breathing out.

        v. Spreading "sparkling stardust": using index finger on one hand, trace each finger of the opposite hand, starting with the thumb: glide up and swooping down through each finger, breathing in on the upward stroke and out on the downward stroke to the pinky finger. Once completed, wiggle the fingers as you blow on them, sprinkling "stardust" throughout the room. Repeat on the opposite hand.

        vi. When the child senses difficulty breathing, explore taking little sips of air in and pushing them out to slow down and encourage fuller breath.

    b. Use imagery while breathing (see "III. Mind" following).

    Add imagery: e.g. inhale by pretending to sip their favorite drink from a straw, exhale it back into the cup; breathing in the ocean breeze through the nose, blowing out the air through their mouth.

iii. Auditory

1. *Voice* – attune to child's vocalizations:

    a. When experiencing pain, match your vocal tone to resonate with child's vocalizations, creating a rhythmic structure to organize their vocalizations.

    b. Have only one person giving directives, especially if in pain, to focus the child's attention.

    c. Try silence or minimal talking if one voice is too much.

2. *Music* – create a playlist of child's favorite music and/or music child and parent find relaxing; this can be anything the child finds engaging, from their favorite and engaging lullaby to a more lively popular children's song.

3. Use instruments such as a rainstick or ocean drum to create to mirror child's vocalizations.

iv. Movement/vestibular

1. Provide active play prior to and at beginning of treatment creating a story related to the child's interests. For example, going on an active beach vacation, providing multisensory descriptive cues to spark the child's sensory awareness.
2. If child is active, initially support movement during pain to support the child's energy level and gradually transition to a full-body "monotonous" imperceptible rocking to calm and regulate the actions.
3. If physical discomfort persists, hold baby in "bucket seat" position with baby's back against adult's torso, adult's arms scooped under baby's knees, with lower limbs relaxed, pelvis suspended; bounce up and down in short, fast, staccato rhythm with accent on upward action matching the rhythm to the baby's vocalization pattern.
4. Once the rhythm is created, add a slight pause after the accent to suggest slowing down the rhythm; as the baby calms, gradually slow down the staccato rhythm, transitioning to swaying side to side to create "monotonous" imperceptible rocking.
5. Check your own breath to make sure it is slow and calm, lengthening your exhale to deepen the calming state.

v. Touch/Proprioceptive

1. Notice the level of tension in the child's body; the child may be tenser when experiencing pain; make sure your body is as calm and soft as possible, breathing evenly.
2. If the child can tolerate touch, engage in foot/leg/belly/whole body massage:

    a. Provide steady touch and/or steady alternating pressure, creating rhythmic pulse e.g. from one foot to the other.

3. If heightened sensitivity to touch during pain:

    a. Withdraw touch if becomes too sensitive.
    b. Provide "touchless" touch by holding your hands slightly above the child's body, sensing their energy and temperature (Reiki approach).

vi. Smell

1. Favorite scents – e.g. lavender oil

vii. Taste

1. Cool sip of water

III. Mind

a. Begin to speak about the treatment prior to coming to hospital discussing multisensory tools that have been helpful in previous sessions. Create image of a "toolbox" of activities you are bringing to support the child.

b. Guided imagery – possible images to build upon during the treatment:

   i. Beach.
   ii. Playing in and hearing ocean waves at the shoreline.
   iii. Take a visit under the sea with a friendly dolphin that comes to help.
   iv. Rise above the ocean waves taking a ride on a hot air balloon up and away floating up into the clouds.
   v. Enter into outer space in a rocket ship, floating in the stardust.

c. Counting breath to gain control.

d. Post-treatment – review activities that helped during the treatment making a plan to add or maintain "(coping) toolbox" for next time.

IV. Emotions (Tortora & Whitley, 2020)

a. Prior to the start of treatment, discuss and plan what the child can have control over.

b. Create playful activities that express child's emotions.

c. Discuss with the child their emotional understanding.

d. Prior to treatment, discuss activities the child enjoys to add to the guided imagery themes:

   i. Create stories that support the patient's emotional state and mood.

e. Keep in mind that the child may become very reticent especially when experiencing pain.

f. Make sure trusting caregivers are present and participant in MSDMT activities:

   i. Discuss with caregiver (and child) specific comforting rituals done at home that can be incorporated into the session such as songs or bedtime rituals.

g. Have favorite objects from home available: e.g. plush toys, blanket, pillow, themed sheets and pillowcase.

h. Fight/flight/freeze reaction during pain:

   i. Minimize the need to verbally respond.

ii.   If able to verbally express:

        1.   Rather than asking the child if she is in pain, drawing focus on the pain, ask: "How are you feeling? Where do you feel this sensation?"

        2.   While breathing with the child, have the parent/medical team exaggerate their breath so the child can hear and feel it.

i.   Ways to address fear/anxiety:

    i.   Be realistic in setting expectations about the treatment.

    ii.   Telling the patient "It is fine. You are OK. It is almost over," when they are not feeling OK, denies the patient's experience.

    iii.   Acknowledge the feeling first – especially if the child is sharing or displaying fear, worry, or sadness – before telling the child everything will be fine. Speak clearly, pausing frequently attuning to child's response. Sample dialogue:

> *Clinician:* "Oh, I understand you are very worried. This really hurts you right now. We are here with you and will keep helping you to make you feel better. Yes, the treatment will make you feel this way."
>
> *Patient:* "I feel like can't breathe."
>
> *Clinician (with caregiver):* "You are breathing well. Let's slow our breath down together."

j.   Periodically provide reminders to slow breath down; verbally and nonverbally describe:

    i.   What is going on; what nurse is doing; other sounds/sensations child is attending to.

    ii.   If child is alert, provide periodic check-ins explaining how they are doing, assuring them the treatment is going well your own actions.

V. Sequence of Activities Example

a.   Prior to treatment, discuss useful rituals/routines that soothe the child, and child's favorite music and play themes; create treatment and play themes around this information.

b.   Playful activities prior to discomfort:

    i.   For infant or toddler:

        1.   Singing favorite playful lullaby tunes or dance-play games especially those that engage the whole body: e.g. "Wheels on the Bus."

2. Peek-a-boo.
   3. Engage in dancing and rhythmic rocking activities for playful engagement and as practice for later use during discomfort.

   ii. For toddler and older child:

   1. Engage in active play and/or dance party with child's favorite music, action/play figures, and/or musical instruments, exploring themes and acting out characters that enable the child to feel empowered.

c. Use of music: a wide variety of genres including parents' favorites may be used that include and go beyond children's music.

d. When discomfort sets in:

   i. Begin to reduce multisensory stimuli related to child's level of sensitivity.

   ii. Singing may continue if child is responding, e.g. parents singing favorite lullaby song such as "Twinkle, Twinkle Little Star."

   iii. Tune into breath, soften singing until just focusing on attuning breath flow to compliment baby's calmer breath

   iv. Caregiver (if available): Cuddle child more firmly if the child can tolerate touch.

   v. For infants, when using bucket seat, securely hold the baby under their knees – adding a pulse to the rock can organize the baby:

   1. Transition to swaying – slowly move baby to shoulder once baby calms.
   2. Make swaying smaller, slower until movement becomes slight, almost imperceptible undulation, side to side.
   3. When calm, remain holding child or place in bed.

Reference

Tortora, S., & Whitley, J. (2020, December 10). Personal communication.

My Body Speaks! Getting to Know Me in the Hospital

PARENTS as PARTNERS

Please help us get to know your child so we can create consistent supportive care together.

Hi! My name is (child's name)_____.

My parents/caregivers' names are_____. Though I haven't completely learned how to use my words to share all my feelings yet, I do understand more than you might think!

We would like to tell you a few ways that I use my body to tell you how I am feeling.

Saying "HI" to me

Approaching me / entering my room:
- ☐ I'm excited to meet you!
- ☐ I look right at you!
- ☐ Eyes become bright!
- ☐ My body gets excited!
- ☐ _____

I get worried easily – notice how I …
- ☐ Stop what I am doing
- ☐ Breath shallowly &/or quickly
- ☐ Won't look at you
- ☐ My body gets tense
- ☐ My body gets agitated
- ☐ _____

I'm shy but want to get to know you. Please understand….
- ☐ I won't look at you at first -but know I'm listening
- ☐ Please pause – approach slowly – talk to my caregiver first
- ☐ Talk quietly with me - give me extra time to respond

Talking to me

I'd love a chat – Notice how I:
- ☐ Orient towards you - become still – focus my attention
- ☐ Suddenly start to move my body
- ☐ Relax and soften my whole body
- ☐ Giggle and smile at you

I'm not in the mood to talk– Notice how I:
- ☐ Tense - look away or immediately at Mommy/Daddy/Caregiver only
- ☐ Cry
- ☐ Turn away - distract myself with my toys/electronic devise

My own special way

_____

I get startled when I don't expect you, (even if I know you). Please….
- ☐ Pause before you come close
- ☐ I feel too sick to look at you
- ☐ _____

My Moods!

My most common feelings are …. (circle all that apply & describe them below)

HAPPY	ENERGETIC!	MAD	SHY	TIRED
PROUD	KNOW WHAT I WANT	SAD	ANGRY	HURTING IN PAIN
CURIOUS	FEELING POWERFUL	SCARED	FRIGHTEN EASILY	STARTLED
TRUSTING		LONELY	SHOCKED	HUNGRY
CONTENT	LOVE SURPRISES	STRESSED	ANNOYED	FEELING SICK
FRIENDLY	HOPEFUL	FRUSTRATED	OVERWHELMED	NEED TIME TO WAKE-UP
CONFIDENT	LOVING	SENSITIVE	WITHDRAWN	
COURAGEOUS	PEACEFUL	CRANKY	SERIOUS	NUMB
SILLY		JEALOUS	WORRIED	SLEEPY
INTERESTED		HELPLESS	BORED	OUT OF CONTROL

These are my own **special body cues.** Watch where my eyes are looking, the intensity of my unique expressions and how I tense, relax, move or **don't** move my body! The feelings I express most are:

When I'm _____ | Eye contact/gaze | facial expressions | body actions

When I'm _____ | Eye contact/gaze | facial expressions | body actions

When I'm _____ | Eye contact/gaze | facial expressions | body actions

My own special mood(s)
_____
_____
_____
 | Eye contact/gaze | facial expressions | body actions

Transitions

The best way to help me when something is about to happen…
- ☐ Let me know what you are doing before you do it, even if you think I'm not listening
- ☐ Tell me what I am transitioning to, and give me a 5 – 10-minute warning
- ☐ I respond best when you _____

What overwhelms me

Sounds
- ☐ Lots of noise in the room
- ☐ Loud sounds - Sudden sounds - beeping
- ☐ Lots of talking all at once
- ☐ _____

Visual
- ☐ Being looked in the eye
- ☐ Bright room
- ☐ Dark room
- ☐ Too many people
- ☐ _____

Touch
- ☐ My body is tender! **Don't touch** me
- ☐ I need warning before you touch me
- ☐ Hot sensations ☐ Cold sensations
- ☐ _____

Smells
- ☐ _____

Taste
- ☐ I need lots of time to take my medicine
- ☐ I **don't** like to eat/drink
- ☐ _____

I 'm very sensitive/get scared when
  Held   Picked up   Moved around in bed
  Please do it like this _____

Ways to help me!

Sounds
- ☐ Talking softly to me
- ☐ I prefer quiet
- ☐ Listening to this music:

  _____

Visual
Your face ☐ Kind/gentle ☐Silly ☐ Calm
- ☐ iPad/electronic device
- ☐ Looking out the window
- ☐ Making a schedule helps me know what to expect

Ways I like to be touched:
- ☐ Hold my hand
- ☐ Hands close but not touching
Massage strokes
- ☐ Pat   ☐ Press   ☐ Glide
- ☐ Circular   ☐ Alternating

} ☐ Gentle
☐ Firm

Massage my:
- ☐ Head ☐ Hand ☐Legs ☐Belly
- ☐ Back ☐ Arms ☐Feet ☐Whole Body

Soothing smells
Use massage cream/oils with a scent
- ☐ Yes   ☐ No   ☐ No cream/oil at all

Eating/drinking *this* makes me feel better

_____

What overwhelms me

Feelings inside - I'm very sensitive/get cranky to these sensations:

- ☐ Nausea
- ☐ Hunger
- ☐ Sleepy
- ☐ Taste of medicine
- ☐ Being cold /hot
- ☐ Needles
- ☐ Bandages taken off / PICC line care
- ☐ Pressure cuff
- ☐ IV Lines
- ☐ NG tube

What triggers me most:

_____

_____

Ways I sooth myself - [Self-regulation]

- ☐ Rub my blanket, shirt collar
- ☐ Vigorously suck my pacifier Stare
- ☐ away - disconnect socially
- ☐ I need to be alone! I will ignore you
- ☐ Keep playing with my toy/iPad/watching movie. I can tune out everything else that is going on
- ☐ Pretend I'm sleeping
- ☐ Rock myself – jump, roll, move around
- ☐ Cozy in my own blanket
- ☐ Cuddling with my favorite stuffy
- ☐ Quietly resting alone

My own special way:

Ways to help me!

I am a cuddler - hold me close like this:

- ☐ Wrap/swaddle me snuggly in a blanket
- ☐ Hold me high up on your shoulder so I can look around
- ☐ Hold me in my feeding position
- ☐ I like to see the whole world all around me. Face me outward against your body
- ☐ **Hold me until I calm down.** I'll show you I'm ready by pulling away/moving my body

Moving around – I need to:

- ☐ Move! Get my feelings out
- ☐ Breath slowly with you. Quiet my body
- ☐ I prefer to be bounced
- ☐ Rocked up & down
- ☐ Swayed side to side   } ☐ Fast ☐ Slow
- ☐ **Let's go!** Take me for a walk

Pacing how you approach me for a procedure

- ☐ Pause! Tell me what you're aboutto do first
- ☐ Talk to me the whole time
- ☐ Counting out loud helps me focus
- ☐ Quiet! As little noise as possible please!

I like to do it myself! Can I help...

- ☐ Give myself the medicine
- ☐ Push the medicine in
- ☐ Do some of the prep tasks
- ☐ Put on the band aid

These are the ways I show you in my body that I am ready _____

Doing it this way helps most _____
_____

Please distract me like this: _____
_____
_____

© 2023 Suzi Tortora and Miri Keren

Uniquely Me!

Special things I want you to know about me *[that may not be so obvious]*

Having fun! My favorites:

Songs
_____
_____
_____

Dance-play / Fingerplay games
_____
_____
_____

Games/Toys/Videos/TV
_____
_____
_____

What make me laugh!
_____
_____
_____

All by myself! Other things I like to do myself:
_____
_____
_____
_____
_____
_____

My favorite people & pets:
_____
_____

Home • Hospital • Home Again:

Routines that help me feel at home wherever I am.

Eating, Food & Schedule
_____
_____

Sleeping / Napping Schedule
_____
_____

What I learned/liked at the hospital for home
_____
_____

Thank you!

Follow the Baby's Lead: Sample Activities for Parents to Engage and Soothe Their Baby

1. **Watch**

   a. Spend some time watching how your baby shifts through different behavioral states: deep sleep – light sleep/drowsy – awake – alert (quiet alert, active alert, vigilant alert) – fussy – crying:

      i. What are your baby's unique ways she lets you know how she's feeling?

2. **Technique**

   a. **Attunement** – match or compliment the nonverbal quality of baby's movements without doing the exact actions. For example: follow the rhythm of baby's leg actions through:

      i. Singing/humming.
      ii. Nodding your head.
      iii. Rocking your body.
      iv. Rocking the crib.
      v. Clapping your hands.

   b. **Mirroring** – match your baby's mood, facial expressions, and actions exactly. For example: Match baby's actions step by step as he looks at you with a broad smile – reaches his left and then right arm out toward you in an alternating pulse – giggles and suddenly lifts his head up, holds it for two counts, and then drops it down.

      i. Build this rapport by making some adjustments:

         • *Mirroring exaggerated* – enhance some aspect of your nonverbal behavior. For example: add a faster beat to your alternating arm pulses reaching and grasping baby's arms/hands.
         • *Mirroring diminished* – softening some aspect of the nonverbal quality. For example: reach your alternating arms out in an undulating flowing pattern as you grasp baby's arms/hands.

c. **Specific movement** qualities and actions to vary/expand your interactions:

    i. *Eye gaze* – look and then look away, providing indirect and direct focused attention in a playful "peek-a-boo" style.

    ii. Timing – play with the timing of your actions, accelerating and decelerating actions and/or your speech.

    iii. *Spatial* – play with how you approach, move with, and move away from baby, creating windy, circular, and straight pathways.

    iv. *Touch and body-to-body contact* – be aware of the quality of your touch such as firm, gentle, long strokes or short patting actions; when holding baby, notice the tension/relaxation and strength of your arms and torso.

d. **Breath awareness** – The quality and depth of your breath in and out (inhale/exhale) and the flow of your breath is a form of communication to your baby, and your baby's breath flow is also a communication about how she is feeling. Steps to bring more breath awareness:

    i. First, notice your immediate breath pattern.

    ii. Take a few comfortable breaths to regulate yourself before you approach your baby.

    iii. Take a moment to tune into your breath periodically while you engage with your baby, and adjust your breath again if you notice you are tense.

    iv. Breath awareness activity to calm/relax:

        • Count the length of your inhale.

        • Exhale one to two to three counts longer than the inhale.

        • Next watch your baby's breath pattern.

        • Synchronize your breath to relate/compliment the pattern of baby's breath flow.

e. **Dance** and **Movement** – notice how your baby responds to each of these actions when in your arms:

    i. Rocking:

        • Create regular accented rhythm.

        • Move baby up and down; side to side; forward and backward.

        • Notice which direction is most calming to your baby.

        • Explore the speed to find which one is most soothing.

    ii. Swaying:

        • Create a fluid flowing swing to your actions without a distinct accented rhythm.

        • Notice how close to your body your baby needs to calm.

- Vary the speed.
- Notice the strength of your hold that best soothes your baby's body.

iii. Dancing to music:

- Watch how your baby is moving their arms or legs or their whole body, and put on a song that matches the rhythm or speed of their actions. It can be a familiar children's song, but it can also be one of your favorites! Chances are your baby will want to connect with your positive, playful excitement.
- Create a dancing dialogue, taking turns leading and following each other's moves, through attunement and mirroring.
- Remember to pace and simplify your actions and give baby time to respond, for he may need a bit more time to process what he is seeing.

e. **Layering the senses** – we have eight senses. Be aware of how many you are engaging you baby in, for they can quickly pile on without our awareness! Think about the rate, intensity, duration of each of these senses:

i. *Interoception* – notice how your baby's internal physical sensations are affecting her mood. What happens to baby's mood when he is feeling hungry, tired or his diaper is soiled?

ii. *Taste* – notice how your baby tells you through her body cues when breast milk, bottle, water, juice, or food satisfies baby's needs; and what body cues tell you she really needs your warmth, comfort or active play instead.

iii. Smell *(your scent)* – when you are not present, leaving a piece of your clothing for the baby to sense, or snuggling with baby's blanket before you go will remind baby of you. Adding essential oils that your baby enjoys, such as lavender, or baby creams with a gentle scent are also soothing.

iv. *Visual* – Follow those eyes! Eye gaze is one way babies tell us they are listening. Notice if your baby is looking at you or away from you. Is the visual contact too much, or soothing? Does your baby prefer to be distracted by a toy or other object? What is the lighting in the room? How does adding or changing the lighting shift your baby's behavior?

v. *Auditory* – Babies respond to their parents' voices talking or singing most. They are also soothed by female vocals. Try lullabies. Notice how your baby responds to music that you enjoy, too.

vi.   *Touch/tactile* – Skin-to-skin contact is very important. There are many ways to touch your baby. Explore which actions your baby responds to most, at what times: long or short stroking, and the strength of your massage stroke.

vii. *Proprioception* – relates to how we sense our body's position in space. One way your baby can sense his body is through pressure. Notice how your baby responses to varying pressure of your hand, or your full body-to-body contact. Try adding and releasing pressure through how you touch, while you hold your baby.

viii. *Vestibular* – this refers to how your baby is sensing her body moving through space. Actions such as rocking and swaying through the room will stimulate this sense. With your baby in your arms explore:

*   How you phrase your actions: *Smooth*, *sway* or *to a beat*.
*   Move in place.
*   Change levels of space.
*   March around the room.
*   "Drop" and swing baby while holding her securely.
*   Dance through the room.

Index

Page numbers in *italics* indicate a figure and page numbers in **bold** indicate a table on the corresponding page.

For Product Safety Concerns and Information please contact our EU
representative GPSR@taylorandfrancis.com
Taylor & Francis Verlag GmbH, Kaufingerstraße 24, 80331 München, Germany